Dorothy Hansine Andersen

John Scott Baird

Dorothy Hansine Andersen

The Life and Times of the Pioneering
Physician-Scientist Who Identified
Cystic Fibrosis

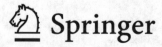 Springer

John Scott Baird
Department of Pediatrics
Columbia University
New York, NY, USA

ISBN 978-3-030-87486-5   ISBN 978-3-030-87484-1   (eBook)
https://doi.org/10.1007/978-3-030-87484-1

This Springer imprint is published by the registered company Springer Nature Switzerland AG
The registered company address is: Gewerbestrasse 11, 6330 Cham, Switzerland

Acknowledgements

Thanks to friends and family who made suggestions after reading an early (very rough) draft, in particular Connie Phillips. Thanks also to Stephen Novak at Columbia University's Archives & Special Collections at the Health Sciences Library, Katie Hafner, and the staff at the podcast series "Lost Women of Science," and Martin Rapp of the New Jersey Natural Lands Trust. This work would have been much more difficult without the support of my wife, Nancy: "don't forget: sweetness."

John Scott Baird

Introduction

As late as the 1930s, infants with lung disease, bulky foul-smelling stools, and inadequate growth in spite of a voracious appetite did not often survive more than a few months. The identification of a new disease—cystic fibrosis of the pancreas, or cystic fibrosis (CF) as we now call it—by Dorothy Hansine Andersen in a 1938 landmark study served to name and define this disease and to ignite academic interest. It was soon appreciated that CF was one of the most common and lethal genetic disorders in the United States and Europe, occurring in one of every three thousand births in northern European populations. In 2020, more than seventy thousand people had the disease worldwide and approximately one thousand patients were diagnosed each year.

Much of Andersen's life remains wrapped in mystery in spite of her importance to the history of medicine in the twentieth century. Whatever renown she enjoyed during her life has diminished, and even some physicians who work in fields she helped define are unaware of her contributions. Controversy about her emerged soon after 1938, as evidenced by comments from a physician colleague: "Dorothy Andersen said that she was the only person in the world who really knew about cystic fibrosis back in the late 1930s and even in the 1940s."

A typical story of CF in the 1930s as reported by Andersen involved an infant whose sibling died at three months of age. She developed "boils" on her arms as a neonate and died with pneumonia at two months of age. At autopsy, Andersen found *Staphylococcus*[1] abscesses in both lungs, and much of the pancreas was replaced by cysts and fibrotic tissue. Many of the patients she identified with this new disease did not survive infancy.

In a series of studies over the first decade following her original description of CF, Andersen was the first to diagnose CF in a living patient, the first to emphasize diet and pancreatic enzyme replacement therapy in CF, the first to successfully treat pulmonary infection in CF with antibiotics, and the first to recognize that CF was a hereditary disease expressed in the manner of a recessive trait. A little more than a decade after her first landmark study of CF, Andersen described heat prostration in CF in another landmark study. This led her to investigate sweat losses of electrolytes in CF with Robert Darling and Paul di Sant'Agnese in January 1953: the findings from this study helped establish a new paradigm for the disease.

---

[1] A type of bacteria.

Unfortunately, Andersen's contributions to CF research and care are often understated, as in a recent book review: "It starts with Dorothy Andersen—the chain-smoking pathologist who recognized the disease's effects on the lungs and pancreas in the 1930s, gave it its name and developed the first diagnostic test." Though correct, this summary neglects many of her contributions to CF care and oversimplifies her understanding of the disease. As it is now nearly a century since Andersen began her medical training and career, and more than fifty years since she died, a more complete appreciation of her contributions is long overdue.

Andersen's accomplishments were not limited to groundbreaking work in CF: she also made contributions to the emerging field of pediatric cardiology, she identified a novel form of glycogen storage disease, and she was involved in some of the first randomized clinical trials of medical therapies in pediatrics. She was widely recognized as an expert in nutrition, a respected pediatrician, a renowned pathologist, a popular teacher, and a brilliant researcher.

Andersen's academic career ran its course at Babies Hospital of Columbia University Medical Center (CUMC) in New York City during the McIntosh Era (from 1931 to 1960): the responsibility and acclaim associated with that setting may be difficult to understand today, but it was considerable. Rustin McIntosh was the Chair of Pediatrics, and his support of Andersen's career was crucial, though they did not seem to share any great friendship. Andersen's colleagues were eclectic and accomplished and a few were truly brilliant; many went on to assume positions of leadership in other academic institutions. Research collaborations at Babies Hospital were frequent during the McIntosh Era, and synergy—in which faculty interactions helped ensure that any accomplishments were greater than just the sum of their individual interests—contributed to their renown. In spite of that synergy, her colleagues also shared a "healthy skepticism," which meant that any opinion was subject to critical review, no matter the source.

Andersen was the victim of gender discrimination, in spite of—or perhaps because of—her academic accomplishments. It is well-known that she was victimized when she was not offered further surgical training after her internship: medical educators were less likely to choose women over men for further training in that era, in part as educators and physicians believed that women were unlikely to remain active physicians as family obligations grew. Though gender undoubtedly played a role in Andersen's career choices, it is more likely that her interest in surgical training was fleeting and cut short in large part by her own illness and a lengthy recovery. Moreover, research she began as a medical student at Johns Hopkins' medical school under several influential mentors helped point her toward an academic career: ultimately, her career as a pathologist at Babies Hospital allowed her the freedom to independently pursue both research and clinical care in whatever direction she chose.

Gender discrimination may take different forms, and some are more insidious than a simple refusal to admit women to further training. Success in the academic setting may engender jealousy, and gender—among other factors—may supply a convenient excuse to use in explanation for actions intended to belittle a successful colleague. Some of the renown she lost over the years may have resulted from colleagues who were able to make light of her contributions because of her gender and comportment; however, she never reacted adversely in any public fashion to criticism, at least insofar as the available records suggest.

She was an only child, orphaned as a teenager, never married, and childless: it is thus a detective's task to learn about her private life. Decades after her death, only a few friends or acquaintances are still available, and very little documentation of her nonprofessional life exists. Interviews with several of Andersen's colleagues (including Michael Katz and Celia Ores) were helpful in that context, as was a visit to the site of Andersen's farm in northwestern New Jersey—her retreat from work. Among the few sources of personal information is an unpublished manuscript entitled "Ahead of Her Time" by Libby Machol,[2] discovered in some papers belonging to one of Andersen's friends.[3] This partial (sixty-seven pages) biography did not cover any of the events following Andersen's 1938 landmark CF study, though Machol did contribute a brief entry on Andersen's life to a biographical dictionary of American women in the twentieth century. Archival materials from Mount Holyoke College, the Alan Mason Chesney Medical Archives of the Johns Hopkins Medical Institutions, and the Augustus C. Long Health Sciences Library at Columbia University were helpful in understanding and contextualizing Andersen's academic and professional life.

Nevertheless, numerous questions about Andersen remain: Who were the important people in her early years? What was her childhood like? How did she make the critical choices which led her to a career in academic medicine? The answers are mostly incomplete or unavailable. But the search for answers illuminates parts of the life of someone with a brilliant, logical mind whose interests were not bounded by what was already known, and whose nature was characterized by a lack of self-importance. She was playful, at times. She also smoked—far too much, especially in the last decade of her life. Smoking for women during this era was viewed as a sign of independence, and a marker of, if not revolt, at least noncompliance with some contemporary social standards.

Controversy about Dorothy Andersen seems to be centered in large part on this streak of independence, and occasionally on her lack of concern about her personal appearance: her hair and clothing were often described as wind-blown and casual, her workplace as disorganized, and her interests outside of work inconsistent with acceptable social norms for a woman. She enjoyed hiking and skiing, canoeing, and other outdoor sports. She enjoyed learning about carpentry and construction: she recruited friends to help build a chimney, replace the roof, and secure a supply of water at her farm. And she did much of it with a cigarette dangling from the corner of her mouth.

---

[2] It is apparent from correspondence in the Archives of Mount Holyoke College that Machol interviewed many of Andersen's friends and acquaintances in the mid-1970s for this work. Machol lived about 2–3 miles away from Andersen's home in Leonia, New Jersey, during the 1950s: Machol and Andersen had several shared social interests, and it would not be surprising if they were acquainted (though there is no evidence of this).

[3] Celia Ores.

Decades after her death, questions related to sexuality might seem important: Why did she remain single and childless? Did she ever live with someone, and if so, what was the relationship? However, these questions have little relevance when considering Dorothy Andersen's career and accomplishments: a nexus of sexuality and career is absent. Andersen and many other gifted women physicians in the twentieth century often led somewhat solitary lives: their success in academic medicine was dependent on devotion to work, whatever their personal inclinations.

In 1952, Andersen was named Pathologist at Babies Hospital and Chief of Pediatric Pathology, having established herself as a researcher, educator, and clinician. Yet she was not universally admired, as noted by Libby Machol:

> Supporters cited the hours she spent helping others with their research projects, her outstanding talents as a teacher, and her consideration for her subordinates. Detractors complained of her disregard of convention and the untidiness of her person and of her laboratory. A tidy mind was important to her; superficial neatness was not.

Detractors did not worry her, as she believed her work—the numerous studies she authored—would continue to speak eloquently of her dedication and insight long after she was gone. But she was gone too quickly: lung cancer claimed her at sixty-one years of age. In the years following her death, many of her contributions have been ignored or attributed to others.

The few remaining examples of Andersen's correspondence, as well as the insights offered by those few still alive who knew and worked with her, suggest that she was a patient, cautious, careful physician uninterested in self-aggrandizement. When she was forced to interact with those who were imperious or dismissive of others, she did not respond with frustration or antagonism; she sought instead to find some compromise, something which would allow collaboration. When conflict appeared inevitable, she ignored them. However, her drive to succeed in academic medicine would not let her give up, even when she was frustrated or ignored, as suggested by Nicholas Christy, another Columbia University physician:

> In great measure [she] had two characteristics that seem self-contradictory: a powerful drive for hard, steady work and extraordinary flexibility. During her research career she successfully reinvented herself two or three times without stumbling, without interrupting the progress of her investigative work.

Andersen's accomplishments were extraordinary: in many ways, she did know more than anyone else about CF in the 1930s and 1940s. Though undervalued, her contributions to our understanding of CF in the 1950s were also significant, and by the time of her death in 1963, many CF patients were surviving into adulthood: Andersen played an important role in that struggle. However, much of her professional career—and almost all of her private life—remain undocumented. A better understanding of her life and career, as well as of her many contributions to the practice of medicine, is long overdue. A recent memorial to William Osler in the *New England Journal of Medicine* by Charles Bryan and Scott Podolsky suggested that:

> Properly taught, the history of medicine can foster among students and practitioners a feeling of belonging and solidarity as members of a profession, a sense of civic responsibility, and ongoing self-reflection.

This biography is offered in that spirit, and it is my hope that it will help stimulate a better appreciation of and interest in Dorothy Hansine Andersen.

Contents

Part I

Life Before Babies Hospital

Time is but the stream I go a-fishing in. I drink at it; but while I drink I see the sandy bottom and detect how shallow it is. Its thin current slides away, but eternity remains.
  Henry David Thoreau, On Walden Pond

Though Dorothy Andersen was born in the South, she always thought of herself as a "Vermonter": stoic, laconic, and a hard worker. These traits frequently ascribed to residents of rural New England appear to define her personality and her career, but only superficially; she was also intellectually gifted, sympathetic to the suffering of others, and self-deprecating. Some evidence suggests that these qualities were present from an early age. It is tempting for a biographer to look for clues in a subject's early life that might help better understand her as an adult, perhaps even suggest what contributed most to her personality and achievements.

However, any attempt to reconstruct Andersen's early life is frustrating, as the few available details only lead to more questions. These mostly unanswerable questions reflect what might seem to many observers to be the hallmarks of a lonely early life: she was an only child whose parents frequently left her to travel to Europe during the summer, she was orphaned as a teenager, and then forced to consider how to finance her college education. Nevertheless, there is no sense of loneliness or despair about her: a sense of accomplishment pervades her academic life, and she seems to have enjoyed friendships and numerous outdoor activities, as well as an expansion of her own cultural and intellectual interests throughout her college career.

Some clues to this apparent paradox may be found in the events of her early life: her parents both died with a chronic illness and Andersen seems to have gracefully shouldered whatever burdens were asked of her, becoming cognizant at a young age of life's fragility. In addition, respect for education and academic accomplishment in her family seems to have been grafted onto the desire to help others, but to do so with an underlying streak of independence. This independent streak helped lead her to a prestigious women's college and then to an elite medical school, followed by a year doing medical research and another year as an intern in surgery (notoriously one of the toughest of all internships); she spent the year following her internship recovering from illness while she toured Europe, sharpening her foreign language skills and "loafing." She then changed course and began to pursue a career in pathology while she completed a doctorate degree.

She rarely complained; rather, it seems she enjoyed it all.

A Beginning

1

During a period of rapid growth in pediatrics and medicine generally, Dorothy Andersen was one of the brightest stars: she was modest, even shy, and her personal background was mostly unimpressive, at least at first glance.

Her father was Hans Peter Andersen: he was born in 1862 on the island of Bornholm in Denmark in the small town of Svaneke. The principal economic activities on this island in the Baltic Sea in the last half of the nineteenth century were granite quarrying and farming, and Dorothy's paternal grandfather – Hans Kofod Andersen – may have been a farmer. In spite of some speculation on the Internet, there is no evidence available to link the author Hans Christian Andersen to Dorothy's family (Andersen is a common family name in Denmark).

Hans Peter had seven siblings, and in June 1868 the entire family emigrated from Denmark: emigration from Bornholm in the last half of the nineteenth century was common, particularly to the United States. Estimates suggest that more than 10% of the Bornholm population left that island for the United States during those years. The Andersen family landed in Boston and then made their way to Danville, Vermont. Hans Peter was then only 6 years old.

He grew up on a farm in Danville [1] adjacent to St. Johnsbury. Conditions on this farm mirrored somewhat conditions his family left behind on Bornholm: chilly winters with lots of snow, rugged terrain with rocky fields, and a reliance on dairy farming. He attended and graduated from St. Johnsbury Academy in 1881, a well-respected local high school that Dorothy as well as other members of his extended family attended years later. Hans Peter went on to study at Dartmouth, where he graduated with a B.A. and Phi Beta Kappa in a class of 250 in 1886 [2] around the same time that his father died during a trip back to Denmark. At his commencement, Hans Peter delivered a "Philosophical Oration: The Philological Study of Modern Languages"; like his daughter, he must have been an excellent, dedicated student and not easily disheartened. It is tempting to speculate that the Andersen family had some broader academic and cultural interests than is suggested by a simple farming

J. S. Baird, *Dorothy Hansine Andersen*,
https://doi.org/10.1007/978-3-030-87484-1_1

background in rural Denmark and Vermont.[1] It is also tempting to speculate that Hans Peter had academic promise and could easily have pursued graduate training, but his family's financial situation didn't permit it. Or perhaps he just felt called to begin helping others, while he was a young adult. Evidence for any of these hypotheses is not available.

Hans Peter began to work for the Young Men's Christian Association (YMCA) shortly after graduation: he served in New York City first and later in Asheville, North Carolina, before advancing to positions of greater responsibility in the International Committee of the YMCA (and various allied organizations). The YMCA is today much less vigorous than formerly: it was originally a popular international movement launched in the mid-nineteenth century with the goal of providing "healthy activities" for young men drawn to cities during the industrial revolution. "Healthy activities" for these young men included a variety of sports and games, the promotion of physical fitness, as well as religious meetings and lectures.

John Mott (a leader of the YMCA as well as the General Secretary of the World Student Christian Federation and the recipient of the Nobel Peace Prize in 1946) was, for most of the last decade of Hans Peter's life, his supervisor. Mott was an evangelist whose interest in the student Christian movement emerged when he was an undergraduate at Cornell and he became closely linked with the YMCA's Student Volunteer Movement for Foreign Missions. He later worked with the World Student Christian Federation (another outgrowth of the YMCA movement) and used that platform to help advance evangelism in the first half of the twentieth century. Hans Peter worked not just for the YMCA but also for the various (Protestant) Christian organizations closely linked to it; Hans Peter and Ethan Colton served as Mott's assistants in the loosely defined "foreign department" of the YMCA during the first decade of the twentieth century (Fig. 1.1).

YMCA World Conferences were held every few years (usually in the summer), beginning in 1855, and the "foreign department" played a significant role in these conferences. Frequent international travel was thus a must for Mott and his assistants: Hans Peter made frequent summer trips to Europe, including in the years 1887, 1889, 1892, 1900, 1902, 1905, 1909, 1910, and 1911 [2]. At least some of these trips were made to coincide with YMCA World Conferences in Norway, France, and Germany, and the rest were likely connected to Hans Peter's work. Colton's career with the "foreign department" grew following World War I and the Russian revolution to include a variety of European relief efforts, mostly under the aegis of the YMCA.

Hans Peter's academic inclinations, as well as his career in a social movement widely considered to embody desirable moral values, suggest a profound intelligence driven by a social conscience to lead a life which had meaning and which emphasized service to others. His work and travel suggest a broad knowledge of European culture and interests. Similar interests were shared by his wife and, later, by his daughter Dorothy.

---

[1] Indeed, several of Hans Peter's siblings also graduated from St. Johnsbury Academy, and one of his brothers – Christian P. Andersen – also graduated from Dartmouth in 1889.

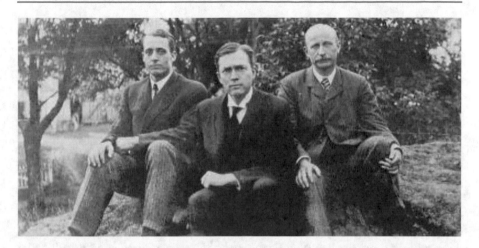

Fig. 1.1 YMCA foreign department officials: Ethan Colton, John Mott, Hans Peter Andersen (L to R). (In the public domain)

Dorothy's mother, Mary Louise (Mason) Andersen, was born in 1868 in Chicago, Illinois. Her family moved to Jersey City, New Jersey, when she was a child, and she grew up there. She may have had an episode of rheumatic fever as a child which left her with a damaged heart [3]. Louise was a descendant of the Wentworth family (colonial governors of New Hampshire) on her father's side. Dorothy's maternal grandparents were Mial Mason (briefly the President of the Board of Education of Jersey City, New Jersey, until his death in 1885) and Lavinia T. (Clark) Mason; both also had family ties to the New England region.

Louise was a graduate[2] of Rockford Seminary (now Rockford University) in Illinois, and she then attended Wilson College in Pennsylvania for 2 years. Both institutions accepted only women: Wilson College advertised itself in 1870 as a place for women "to be leaders, not followers, in society" [4]. Unfortunately Louise was forced to leave Wilson College due to illness,[3] and she did not complete a degree there. The schools Louise chose to attend suggest an interest in some of the reform movements – like women's suffrage and the settlement house movement – beginning to gain momentum in the late nineteenth century. College education for women in the United States was unusual then: it was not until 1950 that 5% of women in the United States had a college degree. At the very least, Louise seems to have been unafraid to consider novel social objectives, and like her husband-to-be, she had a deep respect for education.

---

[2] She likely graduated with a "collegiate certificate" from Rockford, similar to that of the reformer Jane Addams, who attended Rockford a few years earlier (and was awarded a Nobel Peace Prize in 1931).

[3] Likely related to a childhood bout of rheumatic fever, as suggested by Libby Machol.

Louise married Hans Peter in 1892 in Jersey City, New Jersey,[4] and they soon moved to Asheville, North Carolina, with Louise's widowed mother.[5] This small city nestled in the Great Smoky Mountains was a summer resort for many southerners, but the city began to grow quickly around this time, as George Vanderbilt's Biltmore estate was being developed just a few miles to the south. Hans Peter had been working in Asheville for the YMCA since 1889. As his responsibilities in the YMCA (and its allied organizations) gradually increased, travel – both nationally and internationally – occupied more and more of his professional time. Louise often accompanied Hans Peter on his trips to Europe [5], and they also travelled around the southern states on business. But they called Asheville home for most of the first decade of their marriage.

Dorothy Hansine[6] Andersen was born in Asheville on May 15, 1901. She was the only child of Hans Peter and Louise.[7] Asheville during Dorothy's early childhood had both a growing telephone service and a new electric streetcar, though horses were still the most frequently utilized means of transportation, and life still had a rural feel. The novelist Thomas Wolfe was also born in Asheville within a few months of Dorothy, and he described his childhood impressions of Asheville in his novel "Look Homeward, Angel":

> … the smell of hot daisy-fields in the morning; of melted puddling-iron in a foundry; the winter smell of horse-warm stables and smoking dung; of old oak and walnut; and the butcher's smell of meat, of strong slaughtered lamb, plump gouty liver, ground pasty sausages, and red beef; and of brown sugar melted with slivered bitter chocolate; and of crushed mint leaves, and of a wet lilac bush; of magnolia beneath the heavy moon, of dogwood and laurel; of an old caked pipe and Bourbon rye, aged in kegs of charred oak; the sharp smell of tobacco; of carbolic and nitric acids; the coarse true smell of a dog; of old imprisoned books; and the cool fern-smell near springs; of vanilla in cake-dough; and of cloven ponderous cheeses.

It was the portrait of a time and place more closely associated with the nineteenth rather than the twentieth century.

In 1905 Dorothy's family moved to Summit, New Jersey, where they remained for the next decade; Hans Peter had by then returned to work in New York City, in the International Committee of the YMCA. Summit was then and continues to be mostly an upper middle-class community and was also the home of one of Hans Peter's colleagues in the YMCA – John Lovell Murray, who was closely involved with John Mott in the Student Volunteer Movement for Foreign Missions. The small Andersen family purchased some land near the Murray family and built a house [3].

---

[4] Libby Machol notes that they married in Chicago, but the entry for Hans Peter Andersen in Who's Who in New York City and State specifies Jersey City, where Louise was raised and her parents lived.

[5] She died in Asheville in 1894 and was buried with her husband in Chicago.

[6] Hansine is the feminine form of Hans, and it was then a popular girl's name on Bornholm.

[7] An obituary notice for Louise in the St. Johnsbury Republican suggested that Dorothy had siblings who did not survive early childhood; additional evidence supporting this contention is not available, though it is certainly a possibility.

Dorothy later noted that "for the next ten years, suburban winters [in Summit] alternated with long summers spent in Vermont or on the New England coast" [6]. Her visits to Vermont were concurrent with her parents' trips to Europe. Accounts of these trips must have awakened Dorothy's curiosity, as well as a growing interest in European languages and culture: as an adult, she was comfortable reading and speaking German (though perhaps with an accent, according to Celia Ores [7]) – she was also comfortable reading French and Italian – and she travelled as often as she could to Europe.[8] It is likely that Dorothy's independent nature and self-reliance developed in part as an only child whose parents were frequently absent for long stretches of the summer.

Summers in Vermont for Dorothy often included time at Orum Stevens' farm in Danville. Stevens' first wife died in 1880 shortly after giving birth to a daughter – Emma. Stevens' second wife and Emma's stepmother was Mary Christina Andersen, Dorothy's aunt. Though Dorothy was not directly related to Emma or Emma's son – Orum Massey, born in 1910 – both Emma and Orum grew close to Dorothy during her frequent summer vacations at the farm [3].

Dorothy's childhood was clearly different from her father's, as she was raised in a mostly suburban setting during a time of great change: electric lights, automobiles, and telephones were ubiquitous by the end of her childhood. The summer vacations and her father's employment, as well as their residence in the mostly affluent community of Summit, suggest that Dorothy's family did not lack for financial resources; however they were not wealthy. Family resources were earmarked for education and travel in Dorothy's family, reflecting their core values. With few exceptions, that would remain Dorothy's approach as an adult.

In 1909, Dorothy's paternal grandmother, Ane Marie Dahl Andersen, died and was buried in St. Johnsbury, Vermont. Family ties on her father's side to this area of northeastern Vermont continued for several years to exert a pull on the small Andersen family (it is interesting that her mother's family maintained strong ties to Chicago, though Dorothy did not spend much time there). During her summertime visits to Vermont, Dorothy may even have become acquainted with the farm where her father's family lived and worked, as it was likely not far from Orum Stevens' farm. However, Dorothy did not reside in Vermont until the year after her father's death and then maintained her Vermont residence for just a few years until she graduated from Mount Holyoke College. As an adult Dorothy would continue to enjoy the appeal of a rugged New England lifestyle (albeit, not in Vermont), as well as the benefits of international travel.

---

[8] It is possible that Dorothy accompanied her parents on one of their summertime trips to Europe as suggested by Libby Machol, though it could not have been when she was 13 years old as Machol suggested: Hans Peter died prior to Dorothy's thirteenth birthday. In any event, it is easy to envision how such a trip might contribute to Dorothy's lifetime interest in travel and other cultures.

She would, however, always consider herself a "Vermonter"; after all, her father grew up there, and both sides of her family had strong ties to New England. Decades later after her death, a colleague described her character:

> … the only complaints heard from her were the sort of dry, laconic remarks that you would expect from a Vermont farmer contemplating the amount of granite to be removed from a potential pasture. [8]

References

1. Sicherman B, Green CH. Notable American women: the modern period: a biographical dictionary. Cambridge, MA: The Belknap Press of Harvard University Press; 1980.
2. Hamersly LR, Leonard JW, Mohr WF, et al. Who's who in New York City and State, vol. 6. L.R. Hamersly Company; 1914.
3. Machol L. Ahead of her time: a biography of Dorothy H. Andersen, M.D.
4. Wilson College (Pennsylvania). May 27, 2020. Available from: https://en.wikipedia.org/wiki/Wilson_College_(Pennsylvania).
5. Recent deaths: Mrs. Mary Louise Mason Andersen. In: St. Johnsbury Republican. St. Johnsbury; 1920.
6. Dorothy H. Andersen papers. Archives at the Augustus C. Long Health Sciences Library of Columbia University.
7. Ores C. Interview with Celia Ores, J.S. Baird, Editor. 2021.
8. Babies Hospital historical archives. Archives at the Augustus C. Long Health Sciences Library of Columbia University.

Orphaned

One of the most difficult stresses in childhood or adolescence is the death of a parent: Dorothy's father died when she was only 12 years old, and her mother died when she was barely 19 years old. Both parents also had an extended illness prior to death, so that Dorothy had extra demands placed upon her at an early age.

Hans Peter Andersen died on May 5, 1914, at the age of 51 in New Jersey. He was described in a glowing tribute in a publication by the Council of North American Students, itself a contributor to the World Student Christian Federation, as having "tremendous business efficiency" by John Mott,[1] who thankfully had more to say:

> But he had deeper traits. The strongest trait Andersen had, the one I have come to value most of all traits, was his loyalty… He was also genuinely unselfish – the most self-effacing man I have ever been thrown with. I have had the credit of hundreds of things that I do not deserve any credit for, which in the sight of God were due to Hans Andersen. I am not exaggerating; I am understating. Another trait is his genuine spirituality. There is a lot of arrant hypocrisy at times about what we mean by spirituality. Spirituality that is not ethical is not spirituality. Andersen had that which characterizes his race – that transparent frankness and candor and honesty and willingness to die rather than deviate a hair's breadth from what he thought was the truth. [1]

Some of Mott's comments about race and the value of loyalty may seem a bit odd or dated. Nevertheless, it appears that Dorothy's father was perceived as self-effacing, candid, and honest, and he was well-liked by those he worked with: "By his friends, who included, among many others, all his associates, he was counted on as men count on the rising and setting of the sun" [1]. It is a commonplace observation that adolescents may occasionally deplore the personality and behavior of their parents, though they often develop – eventually – a similar character: unselfish, self-effacing, with a paramount concern for the truth, all these are appropriate to use in

---

[1] Chair of the Council of North American Students at that time, and later Chair of the World Student Christian Federation.

© The Author(s), under exclusive license to Springer Nature Switzerland AG 2022
J. S. Baird, *Dorothy Hansine Andersen*,
https://doi.org/10.1007/978-3-030-87484-1_2

describing Dorothy's character as an adult. According to Libby Machol, Dorothy as an adult had mostly happy memories of her father [2].[2]

Interestingly, in spite of his own family ties to Vermont, Hans Peter was buried in Chicago in the same cemetery as his wife's family. There was a memorial service in both Chicago and St. Johnsbury; Mott assisted at the service in Vermont [3].

In 1915, Dorothy and her mother moved from New Jersey to St. Johnsbury [4]. Though by then many of the remaining members of Hans Peter's family had either died or moved away, Dorothy and her mother still had a few ties linking them to this corner of northeast Vermont. The annual summertime visits to Orum Stevens' farm during Dorothy's childhood were treasured memories for her, and she remained close to both Emma and Orum Massey for several years. Dorothy and her mother also knew how her father valued his high school education in St. Johnsbury, and this may have contributed to their interest in moving there. Her mother was by then described as frail and infirm, as she suffered from a chronic illness (likely rheumatic heart disease [2]). As a result, Dorothy took an active role during the move; they left many of their possessions in storage back in Summit [2].

Once in St. Johnsbury, Louise seems to have led a vigorous social life and had many friends, in spite of her chronic illness.[3] She was an active member of the local Congregational church and of the Daughters of the American Revolution, as well as several other local organizations (none of which seemed to interest Dorothy as an adult).

One of Dorothy's few first cousins – Florence Andersen – died in 1916 at the age of 27. She was the only child of Dorothy's uncle Carl Andersen and had grown up in St. Johnsbury. She had also attended St. Johnsbury Academy (as did Dorothy's father and, later, Dorothy). Florence worked for the Young Women's Christian Association (YWCA); unfortunately, she drowned at one of their camps in Michigan.[4] About a month after Florence's death, her father Carl – Dorothy's uncle – who was then living in Dallas, also died and was buried in St. Johnsbury. Though Hans Peter began life with numerous siblings, only a single cousin on Dorothy's paternal side outlived her, and she had very few extended family members on either side of her family as an adult.

Louise and Dorothy lived only a short walk away from the St. Johnsbury Academy, and Dorothy was admitted there without any difficulty (it was the only local high school). Among her classmates, she quickly developed a friendship with several who lived nearby [2]. The Academy is a well-known private, non-profit boarding school; it was the alma mater of Calvin Coolidge and has a long tradition

---

[2] Though it is difficult to credit Libby Machol's assertion that Andersen particularly remembered her father singing "The Lavender Cowboy" to her: a Google entry suggests that this poem/song was first published a decade after Hans Peter's death.

[3] Libby Machol suggested in her biography of Andersen that Louise was then confined to a wheelchair.

[4] She was engaged in Chautauqua work – a social movement with Christian influences which was essentially another overlay to the YMCA. It began in the late nineteenth century with the goal of bringing education, entertainment, and culture to rural America.

of emphasizing college preparatory studies. Historically students living in the town of St. Johnsbury were not charged tuition, and it is possible that this contributed to Dorothy and her mother's move there: after all, Dorothy was the daughter of an alumna of the Academy, and Academy graduates were often admitted to well-respected colleges, like Dartmouth. While the Andersen family was not poor during the first decade of the twentieth century, it is likely that their financial resources were strained or depleted by the end of the second decade; their home in St. Johnsbury was an apartment in a house owned by a Mrs. Boynton [2].

Dorothy's coursework at the Academy included English, history, geometry and mathematics, Latin, German, and chemistry, among other subjects; she did well enough that she was consistently recognized on the honor roll [2]. Dorothy's out-door activities in the winter included snowshoeing, sledding, and ice skating, while she enjoyed hiking, swimming, canoeing, and tennis during other seasons.

St. Johnsbury is the home of the Fairbanks Museum & Planetarium as well as the St. Johnsbury Athenaeum (with its famous collection of paintings by artists of the Hudson River school); both were only a short walk from Dorothy's home. The Museum was the site of additional instruction for local children in native wildlife, including experience in bird-watching: Dorothy apparently benefitted from this instruction [2] and maintained some expertise in bird-watching as an adult.

Dorothy graduated from St. Johnsbury Academy in 1918 [5] and began her undergraduate education at Mount Holyoke College that fall at 17 years of age. However, on May 30, 1920, during her sophomore year, her mother died at the age of 51, the same age reached by her husband. She had been hospitalized for just a day [6], and the death certificate by her physician noted that the cause of death was myocarditis with angina pectoris. It is difficult to know what to make of this: myo-carditis was a non-specific term then used to describe several different types of heart disease. It is likely that Louise's death was related to chronic rheumatic heart dis-ease: death in this setting is commonly the result of either progressive heart failure with valvular damage, an arrhythmia, pulmonary hypertension, or a new infection leading to further damage to the heart valves. However, without more sophisticated medical monitoring and testing or an autopsy, a definitive diagnosis is difficult – if not impossible – to make.

Dorothy had turned 19 years old just a few weeks earlier, and she may have been with her mother at her death [4].[5] Contemplating her mother's illness during the months prior to her death, Dorothy knew where this event would leave her: alone and self-reliant, a college student who needed to pay her tuition and manage her life without family support. Dorothy had a powerful sense of duty which motivated her even during this sad event: she and J. Lovell Murray (her father's YMCA coworker

---

[5]A local newspaper account suggested that Dorothy "was with her when the end came," though Libby Machol suggested that Andersen was notified of her mother's death while at Mount Holyoke, then left for St. Johnsbury, and returned "to college a short time later... [and] that her mother had been buried beside her husband in the Chicago cemetery." A more realistic timeline for these events suggests that Dorothy could not have returned to college "a short time later" and that she would indeed have missed some or all of her scheduled final examinations.

and friend from Summit, New Jersey, who became Dorothy's legal guardian) accompanied her mother's body on its final journey from Vermont back to Chicago [4, 6], where Louise was buried in the Oak Woods Cemetery with her husband, parents, and maternal grandparents. A memorial service was held both in Chicago and in St. Johnsbury. Dorothy would not have been able to return to Mount Holyoke College for at least a week, possibly longer: as final examinations that semester in 1920 were scheduled from June 1 to June 10, she would most likely have needed to make up at least some of her academic responsibilities over the summer.

The effect of losing both parents – as well as several other family members on her father's side and Orum Stevens in 1920, all in little more than a decade – would be overwhelming for most teenagers; Dorothy seemed to draw on deeper reserves. Her independent spirit not only refused to despair, she began a long, steady climb to academic success. Dorothy did not often write about her deepest personal concerns, and when she did she wrote about herself using the third person, perhaps to help distance herself from those concerns:

> The prolonged illness of first one and then the other parent forcibly brought to her attention some of the problems of disease and suggested to her the practice of medicine as a profession. [7]

Her use of the word "forcibly" is curious: rather than being forced to consider a profession, the deaths of her parents actually forced her to confront the lonely future of an orphaned teenager pursuing a college education. Somehow she turned that emotional trauma into a rationale for her pursuit of a career in medicine. Andersen admitted to this emotional trauma in a private conversation, as recounted by Marion Beman Chute to Libby Machol: Andersen told Chute that "having been left an orphan when my mother died was to me such a shattering blow that – having weathered it – no other kind of trouble seems very bad" [2].

With the advances in medical care in the United States which have occurred during the twentieth century, death at the age of 51 is mostly unexpected. Being a personal witness to the death of both her parents at this age did play a significant role in Dorothy's choice of a career in medicine, perhaps including her choice of a particular medical specialty: pathology is dedicated to understanding the causes of disease or death, and her work as a pathologist and medical researcher helped uncover unexpected, life-threatening disease in others.

As her father's family also died off or moved away from Vermont, and following the death of her mother, Dorothy's days in Vermont were numbered: her education would soon take her from Mount Holyoke College to medical school at Johns Hopkins University in Maryland, and she was never again to call Vermont home. Orphaned and on her own as a teenager, she was forced to consider an even more pressing question: how could she hope to support herself while pursuing her studies, and was her dream of medical school a realistic option? Always practical, she embraced part-time work as an undergraduate student as well as scholarship support and part-time work during medical school.

And she made it all seem easy and effortless.

References

1. Irving G. Hans Andersen. The North American Student. 1914;II(9):426–8.
2. Machol L. Ahead of her time: a biography of Dorothy H. Andersen, M.D.
3. Hans Peter Andersen. In: St. Johnsbury Caledonian. St. Johnsbury; 1914.
4. Mrs. Louise M. Andersen. In: St. Johnsbury Caledonian. St. Johnsbury; 1920.
5. Sicherman B, Green CH. Notable American women: the modern period: a biographical dictionary. Cambridge, MA: The Belknap Press of Harvard University Press; 1980.
6. Recent deaths: Mrs. Mary Louise Mason Andersen. In: St. Johnsbury Republican. St. Johnsbury; 1920.
7. Dorothy H. Andersen papers. Archives at the Augustus C. Long Health Sciences Library of Columbia University.

College and Medical School

3

Mount Holyoke College is located due south about 150 miles from St. Johnsbury along the Connecticut River in Massachusetts and is a picturesque college in a semi-rural New England setting. Two of Dorothy Andersen's future colleagues at Babies Hospital – Beryl Paige and Virginia Apgar – also attended Mount Holyoke College: Paige several years before and Apgar several years after Andersen. Though a liberal arts college, it has a strong reputation in science education: "Mount Holyoke inherited an interest in chemistry from the very beginning of the institution" [1]. Laboratory work and undergraduate research have been valuable components of undergraduate science education at Mount Holyoke for most of the twentieth century.

Libby Machol described the expected dress for students at Mount Holyoke College during Andersen's student years:

> During the day, campus wear consisted of pleated skirts (usually navy-blue) with sweaters or middy blouses. For dinner, the girls changed into dresses. For plays and concerts—either on campus or at the Holyoke Community Concert series—evening dress was customary. Girls always appeared in formal gowns at proms…. [2]

Years after Andersen's death, Machol offered this sketch of Andersen as an undergraduate based on reminiscences of her classmates:

> Friends remember her as a "boyish-looking girl with bright flaxen hair and a look of wisdom in her intensely blue eyes. When she smiled, her eyes narrowed to slits, and when she laughed, she'd cock her head to one side, so that she looked almost like a cat." [2]

Andersen's years at Mount Holyoke College (1918 to 1922) encompassed not only her mother's death, but also the Spanish flu epidemic, the end of World War I, and the adoption of the nineteenth amendment to the United States constitution.

The Spanish flu epidemic had an especially dramatic effect on campus life at Mount Holyoke (and may also have helped increase Andersen's interest in medicine): during Andersen's first month of classes in the fall of 1918, "more than a quarter of the College's entire student body of 864 were sickened" [3], though happily only a single student died. Dorothy's hometown of St. Johnsbury was not spared either, as several thousand of its residents fell ill that fall. The end of World War I in November 1918 was an occasion for celebration in spite of the Spanish flu; a war garden established at Mount Holyoke College in 1917 with student support (including student salaries for those who worked in the fields) continued for another year to provide fresh vegetables on campus. The adoption of the nineteenth amendment in 1920 (only a few months after Louise's death) was another joyous occasion at Mount Holyoke, where the pursuit of women's right to vote was widely popular: "Not every women's college was a hotbed of suffragism, but Mount Holyoke was. The faculty was nothing but 'rank women suffragists' one student said" [4]. These public events suggest dramatic change and transformation in student life during Andersen's undergraduate career: how did she deal with the resultant stress?

Quite well: though she was only 17 years old when she began her undergraduate career, she seemed to enjoy everything about her life at Mount Holyoke College. She participated on the debating team (with Marion Beman) and in several sports, learned to ski, and hiked all over the campus and its surrounding woodlands. Her nickname "Andy," used by several of her college friends, suggests the relaxed demeanor of someone unafraid to engage in activities previously characterized as masculine. It is perhaps difficult to believe that she weathered so well the dramatic changes which occurred during her undergraduate years, but she appears to have used them as additional motivation for her own growth and eventual success.

Andersen's undergraduate education was quite broad and included classes in Bible History and Literature, Botany, Chemistry, English, French, German, History, Latin, Mathematics, and Zoology. Though she quickly began to focus her energies on her science classes, she didn't abandon her interest in religion – an interest she shared with her parents: "Laura Wild, who had been a friend of her father's, taught one of the first courses to be offered in any college in which [the] Bible was studied as history rather than theological material" [2]. She also developed a friendship which continued beyond her undergraduate years with Mary Inda Hussey, a renowned researcher in Bible history [2]. Hussey's expertise in the interpretation of Sumerian texts and tablets, among other ancient languages, contributed to her preeminence as a Bible scholar.

After her mother died, Andersen's educational focus at Mount Holyoke College shifted a bit to include more of the courses associated with preparation for medical school: organic chemistry, physics, and comparative anatomy, as well as courses in analytic chemistry and zoology. However her interests remained eclectic, even during her junior and senior years: she took courses in economics, modern philosophy, and psychology.

Andersen majored in zoology and physiology with a minor in chemistry and did quite well in all her courses.[1] She began to acquire interest and expertise in what she

---

[1] Another of Andersen's classmates also majored in zoology and physiology: Miriam Brailey. Interestingly, Brailey grew up in rural Vermont, graduated from Johns Hopkins' medical school several years after Andersen, and also achieved renown with her investigations of another common lung disease of childhood: tuberculosis.

called "laboratory experimentation": she became, in essence, a devotee of the scientific method, in which a systematic exploration of scientific questions is performed using hypothesis testing. The skill and passion she developed for this kind of work would become a hallmark of her academic career. Some of the credit for Andersen's early training as a scientist belongs to two of her teachers: Emma Carr (head of the Department of Chemistry) and Ann Morgan (head of the Department of Zoology). Both of them wrote strong recommendations for Andersen to attend the Johns Hopkins School of Medicine. The Dean at Hopkins responded by writing "In view of what you say concerning her I hope that it will be possible to find a place for her" [5].

Carr and Morgan were well-respected professors with international reputations. Carr suggested years later that the inclusion of research in undergraduate education at Mount Holyoke College was vital: "For myself, the research has added immeasurably to the joy of teaching" [1], helping to explain Andersen's enthusiasm for "laboratory experimentation." Morgan outlined her views on the field of zoology during the time Andersen was a student:

> Modern zoology is no unbranching road. Its paths are yearly becoming more various. To prepare students for the different professions which we have mentioned, we should pursue at least three different directions in the work opened to them: the study of disease-causing organisms, which would open the great field of "medical zoology"; a particular study of responsive behaviors and of the mechanics of the developing animals, experimental zoology; and natural history, the broad knowledge of animals in nature, ecological zoology. [6]

Morgan achieved renown as an early proponent of the study of ecology and conservation: "Now that the wilderness is almost gone, we are beginning to be lonesome for it. We shall keep a refuge in our minds if we conserve the remnants" [7]. Morgan's views were prescient and Andersen seemed to adopt several of them, including a love of conservation with a deep appreciation for the natural world, as well as an understanding that scientific enquiry could never be characterized as an "unbranching road."

The cost of Andersen's undergraduate education was not insignificant: annual tuition was then two hundred dollars, added to another four hundred dollars annually for on-campus housing.[2] She did not receive any scholarship help [8], though she was a very good student. It is possible that she inherited some financial resources, but they were not sufficient to cover all her expenses. Several years later when Andersen's colleague Virginia Apgar attended Mount Holyoke College, Apgar supported herself and helped pay for her education by working in various campus jobs including "the college library, waiting on tables, and catching stray cats for comparative anatomy classes" [7]. Andersen took advantage of similar opportunities: "The Biology professor, noting her [Andersen's] interest and ability, offered her a job as a lab assistant, to set up materials for student experiments" [2]. She also worked as a camp counselor during summers, and it is quite possible that she worked in the war garden, or caught some cats, or performed any number of other odd jobs

---

[2] In 2020, this would be equivalent of just under $10,000 per year.

on campus during the school year. The summer of 1922 following her graduation she worked as a camp counselor in Altamont, New York, with her classmate Marion Beman [2]:

Andersen suggested in 1923 that she did owe the college some money:

> Medical school is expensive, and I don't feel able to pay anything until I get out. I have already pledged my 305, and expect to pay it the first year after graduation, which will be 1926–27. [8]

There is no record for when she finally paid the $305 or what that might represent (while it could represent student debt, it is more likely that she made a pledge for this amount to the Alumni Association after graduation). In any case, during the decades which followed Andersen never neglected to keep the Alumni Association informed of her activities. It is notable that she retained many of the attitudes and interests she developed at Mount Holyoke throughout her adult life: she clearly felt a strong attachment, a strong debt that wasn't just financial, to those associated with her undergraduate education.

On the other hand, Andersen's independent streak meant that she was never shy about offering contrarian opinions. In 1960 toward the end of her life, she completed a Mount Holyoke questionnaire, and in reply to the question "If you were entering college today, would you choose Mount Holyoke?" she answered "No" [8]. She had, by then, decided that a coeducational college was a better choice.[3]

In spite of her financial worries and concerns about student employment, Libby Machol reported [2] that Andersen as an undergraduate still found the time and resources to take a number of vacations, mostly with her classmates: to New York City, to the Murray home in Summit, to the Massey farm in Vermont, and on overnight camping jaunts around Mount Holyoke College. One of these vacations to the Massey farm affirmed Andersen's sense of humor:

> One Easter vacation, she [Andersen] brought her roommate, Edith Knight. The two decided to play a practical joke—an April Fool prank—on the hired man. They arranged a wastebasket loaded with cushions, balls, and crumpled newspapers so that its contents would tumble down on him when he pulled the cord to switch on the electric light in his room. The hired man was furious. He delivered himself of a few sharp words about "smart young 'uns" before setting off to walk the miles into town, leaving the evening chores unfinished. Dot took over and had a fine time cleaning out the pig pen and watering the horses. Edith helped as long as she could, but finally had to slip off to the seldom-used "best room" for a nap. Dot woke her in time for the lavish country dinner she'd helped cook after the barn chores were finished. [2]

Missionary work by Mount Holyoke College alumni was common during the college's first century, in part reflecting its strong Protestant background. Andersen became firmly committed to becoming a doctor, while she was an undergraduate, and after joining the Student Volunteer Movement for Foreign Missions (SVMFM), she began to consider service as a missionary doctor in Africa following medical

---

[3] In that same questionnaire, she also identified "integration, state medicine, education" as political, cultural, or social problems of concern.

school [2]. SVMFM was closely linked to the YMCA, and John Mott was among its earliest leaders. Andersen's father had also been involved with the SVMFM, as was Ethan Colton and J. Lovell Murray (Lowell became Andersen's legal guardian after her mother's death). Many of Andersen's classmates and friends were also members, occasionally even officers, of the Mount Holyoke College chapter of the SVMFM, including Marion Beman, Edith Knight, Louise Eby, and Marion Nosser. With these personal connections, it is not surprising that Andersen gravitated toward the idea of missionary work.

Andersen's senior yearbook photo suggests calm determination and perhaps a hint of mischievousness.[4] She graduated in June 1922 from Mt. Holyoke College with a B.A. [7] (Fig. 3.1).

Her application for admission to Johns Hopkins included a request for "works you have read in Latin," and she responded with "Caeser's Gallic Wars, Cicero (7 orations), Virgil's Aeneid (4 books), Ovid- selections from Metamorphoses, Plautus (2 plays), and selections from the poets": an impressive list. She also noted that she had modified her coursework during her last undergraduate semester to include a

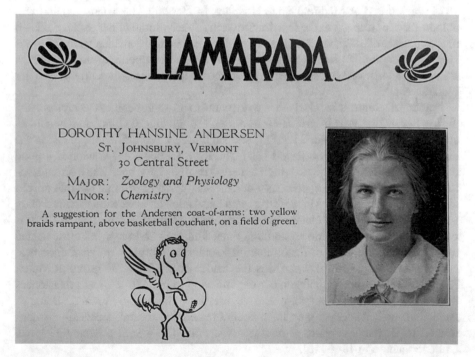

Fig. 3.1 Yearbook entry for Dorothy Andersen at Mount Holyoke College, 1922. (In the public domain)

---

[4] Since the sport of basketball was invented at a YMCA facility in Massachusetts around the time her parents were married, it is tempting to speculate that the sport may have had some connection for Dorothy with her father.

course in German reading and grammar; she further noted on her medical school application that she could read both French and German. She was notified of her admission to Johns Hopkins School of Medicine in July 1922; she began first year coursework in October. There were five other women in her medical school class.

Andersen received some scholarship assistance (a research fellowship from the Henry Strong Denison Medical Foundation) for several years at Hopkins. During the summer of 1923 following her first year in medical school, she worked as "Camp Director" in Franklinville, New Jersey [8]. Later that summer she noted in a letter to the registrar: "I am still poor, and I still want a job next year in or around the hospital or medical school that would pay something towards my expenses. Has anything at all turned up?" The registrar replied:

> My dear Miss Andersen: … Things are very quiet on the Patapsco at present. I feel confident, however, that something may turn up before you are a week in the school, in which event I will see that you are given an opportunity to avail yourself of it. Do not fail to report in the fall and continue the good work which you have already started. [9]

There is no record of her employment during that school year, but in the summer of 1924 she worked at Medfield State Hospital, in Harding Massachusetts, and was able to forward a check to the registrar covering at least some of her expenses. Then in the summer of 1925, she spent over a week being treated for sinusitis in the Johns Hopkins Hospital [8] and spent most of that August recuperating in Entrelacs, a small town northwest of Montreal [8]; summer employment apparently passed her by that year.

Andersen's interest in missionary work came to an abrupt end in December 1923 during her second year in medical school: while attending the ninth annual conference in Indianapolis of the SVMFM, she submitted a preliminary application for missionary work but was rejected [2]: "The form [application] contained a good many theological questions, to which her answers must have been less than satisfactory" [2]. Like many young adults, Andersen was then reexamining the role of religion in her life, and Libby Machol suggested that Andersen's rejection for missionary service marked a definite change in her attitudes toward organized religion [2]; it is worth noting that beginning around this time, Andersen no longer felt close or tied to any particular church or denomination.[5] Andersen's Mount Holyoke classmate and close friend Marion Beman was the leader of the SVMFM group at Mount Holyoke College during their senior year and went to India in 1924 as a missionary for the Congregational Church, where she met her (missionary) husband.[6] Beman's friendship with Andersen may have been strained for several decades – perhaps related to Beman's support of missionary service [2] – until a Mount Holyoke College reunion in 1948 [10].

---

[5] Andersen's response to a 1923 Mount Holyoke College Alumnae Questionnaire indicated she was a member of the Presbyterian church, though she left later requests for religious affiliation blank. By 1936 she answered the same request by describing herself as "agnostic."

[6] Another Mount Holyoke classmate and friend – Marion Nosser – served as a missionary in Turkey from 1925 through 1927; she later made her home there as a teacher.

Andersen's rejection for missionary service by the very group that her father and his associates supported might suggest that Andersen would then have felt less connected, less influenced by her father's memory and by his concerns generally. However that is unlikely: as John Mott observed about Hans Peter Andersen, he "had that … transparent frankness and candor and honesty and willingness to die rather than deviate a hair's breadth from what he thought was the truth"; so did his daughter share that same frankness, candor, and honesty. Mott's recognition of the ethical nature of Hans Peter Andersen's "genuine spirituality" could also be applied to the daughter: neither one owed allegiance to organized religion for their spiritual life, and both possessed an ethical approach which prevented each of them from deviating "a hair's breadth" from their perception of truth. Though Andersen's father had died nearly a decade earlier, Andersen's ethical concerns as an adult seemed to echo those of her father.

Also in 1923, Andersen began her research career studying the female reproductive system in different animal species in the Hopkins laboratory of Florence Rena Sabin, whom Andersen described as "a dynamic teacher" [8]. Sabin had been an intern under the legendary William Osler [11] and was the first woman to be a full professor at Johns Hopkins School of Medicine [12]. Sabin was originally an anatomist: for much of her career at Hopkins, she taught in the Department of Anatomy. A century later, there are many fewer anatomists in medical schools, in large part because anatomists were ultimately successful at providing a good understanding of the structure-both gross and microscopic-of organs and tissues in the body.

Sabin suggested that Andersen focus her research during medical school on the lymphatic vessels associated with the female reproductive system, and Andersen's work in this field in 1923 marked the beginning of her academic career. Andersen continued this work for several years, eventually broadening her focus to include the changes which occur in the female reproductive system and other endocrine glands during ovulation.

Sabin left Hopkins in 1925 to accept a position as head of the Department of Cellular Studies at the Rockefeller Institute in New York City where she was the first woman to achieve membership (equivalent to the rank of professor). Sabin was a renowned physician with expertise in several fields, including embryology, immunology, and public health, and she enjoyed a long career full of honors: the authors of a biographical memoir published by the National Academy of Sciences suggest that "By her [Sabin's] example she did more than any other person to open the careers of scientific investigation in laboratories, medical schools, and hospitals to women" [12]. Sabin's career also suggested the direct transfer of an academic heritage: from Osler to Sabin to those Sabin mentored, including Andersen. It would then be up to Andersen, among others, to help ensure that this heritage didn't die out.

George Streeter and George Corner, both of them renowned anatomists who also studied at Hopkins, helped mentor Andersen with her research after Sabin left Hopkins to join the Rockefeller Institute. Andersen's research was published over several years, both while she was a student and after she graduated: she was an exceptional student, and she was mentored by several of the brightest stars in academic medicine.

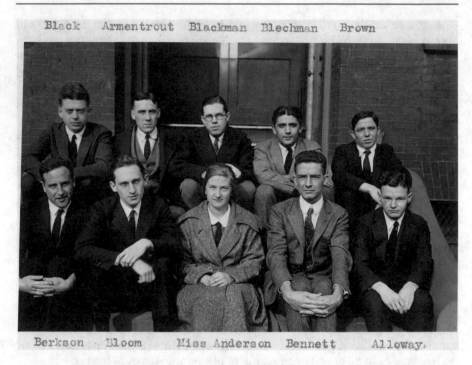

Black   Armentrout   Blackman   Blechman   Brown

Berkson   Bloom   Miss Anderson   Bennett   Alloway.

Fig. 3.2 Dorothy Andersen as a senior medical student (front row, center) with nine of her colleagues. (Courtesy of Alan Mason Chesney Medical Archives of the Johns Hopkins Medical Institutions)

However, as a senior medical student in October 1925, Andersen was still ambivalent about her future: she considered an internship in internal medicine in 1926 at New Haven Hospital,[7] but she kept postponing the decision, and she still had not decided on a career choice by the time she graduated [7]. Finishing the work she had started in Sabin's lab was certainly a priority, but how could she do this during an internship? She could perhaps procrastinate by taking a lower-level academic position without clinical responsibilities for a year or two, completing her research, and make a decision then. Since the death of her parents, she had been relentless in her pursuit of education and academic excellence and showed no signs of fatigue or boredom or a lack of ability. In spite of an illness and hospitalization during medical school, Andersen greatly enjoyed her medical education and began to see a future for herself in academic medicine. Sabin was an early role model for Andersen, and Sabin's career suggested a similar possibility for other exceptional women unafraid of hard work. It would take time, but Andersen believed she had plenty of that.

---

[7]Andersen's classmate at Hopkins – H. Houston Merritt – began his training at New Haven Hospital following graduation. He served later as the Dean of Columbia University's College of Physician and Surgeons at the end of Andersen's career.

At 25 years of age, she was still young, and as a newly graduated doctor, she had reached a major goal: it was time to sit back and survey the landscape, consider her future, and keep her options open (Fig. 3.2).

She was flexible.

References

1. Carr EP. Research in a liberal arts college. J Chem Educ. 1957;34(9):467.
2. Machol L. Ahead of her time: a biography of Dorothy H. Andersen, M.D.
3. Lammel O. Campus under quarantine. Mount Holyoke Alumnae Quarterly. 2015;99(1):28–31.
4. Lepore J. The secret history of wonder woman. Vintage; 2015.
5. Rustin McIntosh papers. Archives at the Augustus C. Long Health Sciences Library of Columbia University.
6. Morgan, A. An undated letter, circa 1921–1922. 1921.
7. Sicherman B, Green CH. Notable American women: the modern period: a biographical dictionary. Cambridge, MA: The Belknap Press of Harvard University Press; 1980.
8. Dorothy H. Andersen papers. Archives at the Augustus C. Long Health Sciences Library of Columbia University.
9. Dorothy. H. Andersen papers. Alan Mason Chesney Medical Archives of the Johns Hopkins Medical Institutions.
10. Miller MP. History of Andy's farm, M. Rapp, Editor. 2013.
11. Dawson P. Dorothy in a man's world. North Charleston: CreateSpace Independent Publishing Platform; 2016.
12. McMaster PD, Heidelberger M. Florence Rena Sabin. Biographical memoirs. National Academy of Sciences; 1960.

False Start

4

After medical school graduation in 1926, Dorothy Andersen accepted a position as Assistant in Anatomy at the University of Rochester School of Medicine [1, 2]: she assisted George Corner [3] – a colleague both of Florence Sabin and George Streeter. Sabin, Corner, and Streeter all shared a Hopkins bond, and each became a respected leader in related fields of academic medicine.

Sabin was mentored by Franklin Mall while she was a medical student at Hopkins, and later by William Osler while she was an intern; she then mentored Corner while he was a medical student. Streeter was also mentored early in his career by Mall – whom he succeeded as Director of the Carnegie Institution of Embryology and Corner eventually succeeded Streeter as the Institution's third Director. Corner was keenly interested in defining the physiology of ovulation and worked extensively with animal models, particularly pigs; his work helped establish the role of the corpus luteum and progesterone in female reproduction. These three anatomists had been quick to recognize Andersen's academic promise and were in a position to help her begin to achieve success.

An anatomist's work – focused on the finest details of anatomy in order to help reveal the relevant physiology – might appear unexciting, even a bit tedious at times. However Andersen didn't see it that way: "The fascination of laboratory research was detrimental to faithful attendance at classes [4]," while she was a medical student (and even earlier as an undergraduate). The meticulous, rational approach she adopted with her early work on female reproduction stayed with her throughout her career.

A prolific correspondence with Streeter regarding several of the details in her early studies on female reproduction offers some insight into Andersen's work as a budding anatomist. In one of her 1927 manuscripts [5], she was hoping to provide a complicated figure to show the relationship of the lymphatics draining the fallopian tube of a sow at different points along its course, but in three dimensions: nearer to the uterus, she wanted to show the prominent lymphatic sinuses on the inner surface – or mucosa – of the tube. She made a preliminary sketch (Fig. 4.1) to emphasize these spatial relationships: on the far left she tried to show prominent lymph

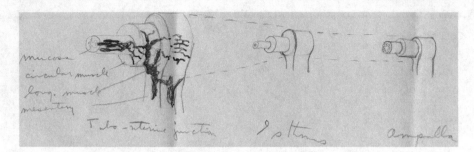

Fig. 4.1 Andersen's sketch in her correspondence with Streeter regarding her 1927 study on lymphatics of the fallopian tube. (Courtesy of the Alan Mason Chesney Medical Archives of the Johns Hopkins Medical Institutions)

sinuses near the mucosa extending along the long axis of the fallopian tube at the tubouterine junction.[1]

The renowned medical illustrator James Didusch at Hopkins provided several figures in an attempt to render these spatial relationships for Andersen's study.

In Fig. 4.2 (upper left) Didusch showed the complete Fallopian tube and associated serosa, to which Andersen's sketch of the cross sections at different points correspond. In Fig. 4.2 (lower left) he portrayed in microscopic cross section the prominent lymph sinuses (in blue) in the mucosa layer of the fallopian tube at the tubouterine junction, while in Fig. 4.2 (lower right), he portrayed the lymph vessels (again in blue) in the mucosa layer of the ampulla of the fallopian tube:[2] these last vessels take a different course that Andersen wished also to emphasize (but did not include in her sketch), running perpendicular to the long axis of the fallopian tube along the inner mucosa layer and then emptying into slightly larger lymph vessels running along the long axis of the fallopian tube in the circular muscle layer.

Though this meticulous analysis might seem to be of limited interest, the precision and care she brought to this research suggest a kind of dedication that would be quite helpful to her later; this was, for the most part, the principal component of the academic heritage she received from Sabin. However, her rational and intuitive nature suggested some practical application of this knowledge: she speculated that an infection of the uterus or fallopian tube might be absorbed via these lymph sinuses and vessels before reaching the ovary or the peritoneal cavity and that the lymph vessels of the ampulla – which seem to reach into the lumen of the fallopian tube like tiny fingers – might be particularly important in that context.

Andersen recalled a pathology specimen at Hopkins from a patient with acute salpingitis,[3] in which the lymph vessels of the ampulla were packed with white blood cells secondary to an infection: she suggested that anatomic structure and physiologic function were closely related, as the lymph vessels reaching into the

---

[1] The transitional section of the fallopian tube as it enters the uterus.

[2] A section of the fallopian tube closer to the infundibulum and ovary.

[3] Inflammation of the fallopian tube.

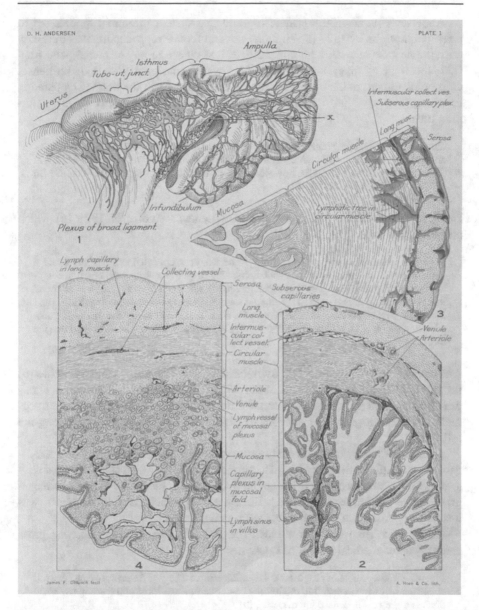

Fig. 4.2 James Didusch's illustration for Dorothy Andersen's 1927 study on lymphatics of the fallopian tube [5]. (In the public domain)

lumen of the tube were helping to resolve the infection before it spread any further upstream. A similar approach linking anatomic detail with physiologic response was used by Andersen throughout her research career. She ended this detailed discussion with an unusual comment for an academic study: "It is a matter worth considering, at any rate" [5], seeming to speak directly and a bit informally to the reader.

Andersen's work on the female reproductive system in animal models led to three publications by 1927 [5–7]: more work on female reproduction was to follow over the next decade. Though appearing at first glance to be somewhat pedestrian (like the work of many anatomists), there were occasional flashes of brilliance. Corner later noted in his book "Hormones in Human Reproduction" [8] a paradox involving how eggs are transported from the ovary to the uterus via the fallopian tube:

> the oviducts [or fallopian tubes] of different species of animals are of very different lengths, and yet with only a few known exceptions, the eggs make their journey through them in about the same time… The cilia, however, certainly do not beat that much more rapidly [in animals with longer oviducts]. [8]

He then discussed the results of one of Andersen's studies in 1927 [6] which addressed this paradox:

> A former colleague of mine, Dr. Dorothy Andersen, once collected at a packing house a very large number of oviducts of swine containing eggs. She cut up each one into 5 segments and examined each segment separately to see whether it contained eggs. She found that it is common to find eggs in the middle segments, but rare to find them in the first and in the last parts of the tube- in other words, the eggs are rushed through the first fifth, transported very slowly through the middle stretch, and then hurried through the last part into the uterus. [8]

Andersen actually collected 168 oviducts (or fallopian tubes) from 84 swine [6] for this investigation. As a result of her work, Corner noted that academic attention shifted from the cilia to differential muscle contractions of the various segments of the fallopian tube in order to explain the movement of eggs along the fallopian tube.

Andersen's research at this early point in her career suggested a lively intelligence and imagination and affirmed her great capacity for work, as well as an ability to make novel observations. It is notable that Corner referred to Andersen, a recent graduate, as "a former colleague": the esteem in which he held Andersen was instructive – Andersen's mentors valued her contributions.

At the same time that she pursued her research, she was also teaching gross anatomy at the medical school in Rochester:

> In an article in a journal of progressive education entitled *The New Student*, Joseph Chassell wrote the following description of Dorothy Andersen's class: 'Most of the group work and discuss together—it is more fun that way. [9]

She was quickly becoming a respected anatomist and researcher, as well as a popular teacher, all in the tradition of her Hopkins mentors.

Corner later wrote a memoir about Streeter, describing his research methods and their limitations, but in the end affirming the high value placed upon an anatomist:

> Streeter was never an explorer of the rough and ready kind. His work contains few totally novel observations, but he possessed supreme ability to take up imperfectly understood

phases of embryonic development, refining, integrating, and accurately depicting them. His predilection for this kind of work was founded, no doubt, upon the mental characteristics that went with his exceptional talent for accurate drawing. [10]

It is this tradition of academic excellence, represented by renowned and dedicated anatomists like Streeter, Corner, and Sabin, that Andersen was preparing to join in 1926. The academic heritage that William Osler passed onto Sabin was not a secret handshake or a secret book of medical knowledge: it was a reliance on hard work coupled with a broad knowledge of biology, used to help define and eventually treat human disease; it is, of course, true that insight and imagination would be essential in order to make the "novel observations" which characterize the stunning advances in medical knowledge of the twentieth century. Osler made frequent use of detailed case studies or case series of patients with a particular disease in order to help explain the disease process, that is, the pathophysiology. Andersen's similar reliance on her recollection of a patient with acute salpingitis in order to better understand the anatomy and function of lymph vessels in the female reproductive tract illustrates how she continued that practice.

Andersen's academic training up to that point had prepared her for a productive career in academic medicine, but she was not yet quite ready to follow that path. Perhaps she recognized in herself a tendency both to novelty and precision; it is likely that a year of working tediously as an anatomist and gradually coming to terms with the slow pace of research and publishing in academic medicine helped to push her in a slightly different direction, at least transiently: her independent streak was about to assert itself in a minor career detour, or false start.

While working in Corner's lab, Andersen considered further clinical training: she decided to begin an internship in surgery in the summer of 1927 at the University of Rochester's Strong Memorial Hospital. She interrupted, at least temporarily, her research interests in the female reproductive system as well as her own academic inclinations. Years later Andersen noted that she originally "had plans for a country practice if the academic world wouldn't have me" [4]. In reality, it was the other way around: she deserted the academic world to follow the lure of surgical training. Her remark, characteristic of her modest and unassuming demeanor, was belied by the response of one of her mentors: a letter from Streeter in September 1927 expressed the surprise engendered by her choice of a surgical internship, "I am quite shocked that the lure of the operating room has wrecked [sic] havoc with your plans. You may, however, become tired of this and return to the fold at some future time." Andersen's reply in late October 1927 was informative: "I'm sorry to disappoint you by deserting to the surgeons, but it isn't impossible that the future will find me returning to the fold. This year is certainly an interesting and strenuous, if not entirely a pleasant experience" [4].

Very few women were admitted to surgical training in the United States during the first half of the twentieth century, and fewer still were able to finish that training and establish a surgical practice. In retrospect, it is clear that Andersen's pursuit of surgical training was valuable to her, if not entirely consistent with her previous educational efforts. Surgical training was the first choice for several other exceptional women medical school graduates around the same time: Virginia Kneeland in 1923 (the first woman accepted into a surgical internship at Columbia University) and Virginia Apgar in 1933. These women were intellectually gifted like Andersen, members of a new generation just then being admitted into the male bastion of academic medicine, including the even more exclusive bastion of surgery. Apgar left surgical training for anesthesiology,[4] while Kneeland persisted for several years in an academic surgical practice.[5]

Andersen was denied further training as a resident in surgery by "hospital policy" (and must have known this when she started); whenever hospital policy was nebulous, social attitudes were not. Medical educators and physicians believed that valuable training would be "wasted" on women who were unlikely to remain active in the profession as their family obligations grew.[6] In addition, the competitive, aggressive nature of many surgeons, as well as the physical and emotional strain of many operative procedures, did not seem to fit well with social attitudes then current regarding the female gender. Such considerations from nearly a century ago now seem simple-minded, but they were no less real at the time. This episode was a clear example of gender bias, though Andersen's subsequent career path did not reflect frustration or deep disappointment, and she seemed to have no regrets about her year of internship training.

Indeed, her remark that her internship year was "interesting and strenuous, if not entirely pleasant" appears to be a coded approval, as it suggests that any potential benefits were worth the discomfort. She did not complain or blame others for the lack of further surgical training opportunities. Ultimately, it is likely that the internship in surgery helped prepare her for future challenges: she learned how to cope with stressful situations, she developed a bit more self-confidence, and she learned to rely more on her own judgment. Moreover, she added an intense clinical awareness to her understanding of physiology and her training at Hopkins as a meticulous anatomist. Though she was always drawn to laboratory investigations throughout her career, she was also drawn to patient care, and her internship helped her begin to recognize that need.

---

[4] Allen Whipple, the Chair of the Department of Surgery at Columbia University, suggested to Apgar that anesthesiology would be "more suitable" for women. However, gender bias apparently was also an issue in her pursuit of training in anesthesiology. Perhaps to his credit, following Apgar's training in anesthesiology, Whipple was supportive of her return to CUMC as an attending anesthesiologist.

[5] Kneeland had a surgical practice for several years at Columbia University Medical Center (CUMC) after her training but then switched to surgical pathology and achieved renown in this field (under her married name: Frantz).

[6] Years later on November 5, 1939, the Babies Hospital Medical Board was asked to express its opinion about the appointment of women interns to the intern staff. "It was the consensus of the Board that so long as women were accepted in medical schools, the first class hospitals were almost obligated to accept them for training. Positions on the Babies Hospital staff should be available." This action by the Board came during the McIntosh Era, 22 years after the first women were accepted at Columbia University's College of Physicians and Surgeons (of note, Babies Hospital accepted women as physicians-in-training beginning with its original founding by women, long before its association with Columbia University).

Nevertheless, the frustration and difficulties inherent in a year of surgical internship (taken up originally with the intoxicating if somewhat romantic image of a country medical practice utilizing surgical skills) were eventually complicated by illness: when she fell ill at the end of her internship year, that was indeed the end of her surgical training. And she was ill: she was told to take time off and ended up spending a year in Europe.[7] In an autobiographical sketch years later she wrote:

> At the end of this time, she [Andersen] had a prolonged attack of infectious hepatitis, which she considers to have been a most fortunate circumstance, since it resulted in orders to cease work for a year. Since loafing in Europe was much more interesting and no more expensive at that time than convalescence in the U.S.A., she spent the following year in France and Italy, learning the languages, looking at pictures, pursuing her hobby of sketching and being laid up in friendly but not always comfortable little hotels at odd places by recurrences of jaundice. [4]

Exposure to blood-borne pathogens like hepatitis viruses is a major risk for surgeons, particularly during training when one's skills are still developing. An incidental sharp injury (e.g., a needlestick or a minor cut from a scalpel) during surgery could easily have exposed Andersen to a hepatitis virus, explaining her illness.

Despite Andersen's obvious interest in and enjoyment of "loafing in Europe," it is important to place this trip in context: she was a young woman on a solo adventure, and she was not healthy.[8] She had no family or close friends monitoring her progress, no one to turn to in the event of an emergency. The degree of independence she manifested was remarkable. Her surgical internship seems to have left her with the confidence to confront all kinds of potentially uncomfortable situations during a time when a woman's place in society was still restricted.

Andersen's European tour gave her time to sketch, learn some Italian, and brush up on her French and German, as well as think about her career goals: she realized that an academic setting in which she could continue both to pursue her studies on female reproduction and refine her anatomic skills was most appealing. Though a country practice might also be appealing,[9] it could not satisfy her: she felt the need

---

[7] It is intriguing to note that in addition to Andersen, at least five individuals mentioned in this biography also spent an extended period of time in Europe between 1928 and 1930: Rustin McIntosh, H. Houston Merritt, Geoffrey Rake, Abner Wolf, as well as the novelist Thomas Wolfe. At least for those interested in a career in academic medicine, Europe remained an important destination during the first few decades of the twentieth century.

[8] An alternative explanation for Andersen's European trip in 1928 was offered by Celia Ores in 2021: near the end of Andersen's life, Ores remembered that Andersen told her she went to England following her surgical internship in order to meet the family of a young man she planned to marry, that she became sick on the voyage, and that she was hospitalized for hepatitis on her arrival in London. According to Ores, Andersen then started to smoke. In the absence of confirmatory evidence, it is difficult to know how to interpret this.

[9] Early in 1930 she obtained a license to practice medicine in the state of Vermont. It appears she was covering her bets, ensuring that she could pursue a "country practice" there if she wished. Among the various state licenses to practice medicine she obtained over her career, she preserved only her Vermont certificate in her files. It is tempting to suggest that she did so in part to remind herself of the road not taken.

to somehow bring her studies on female reproduction which she had started at Hopkins to a meaningful conclusion, and she recognized that a career in pathology might also offer interesting research opportunities. Presbyterian Hospital – just then emerging as a major component of Columbia University's new medical center – had an opening in pathology, and Columbia University had a doctorate studies program which could be easily adapted to her research interests. After an absence of a few years, she was about to resume the academic medicine track she had been on at Hopkins, absent the Hopkins mentorship.

A reboot of her career with a focus on pathology was an interesting choice after her false start in surgery. There is no evidence that she felt regretful about not choosing to get training in internal medicine or about the illness she suffered following her internship. She was eager to reinvent herself as a pathologist, and she seemed to understand that all her knowledge and training up to that point would eventually prove useful.

Moreover, she appeared to enjoy all of it: her education, her research, even her false start in surgical training; and she certainly enjoyed her European tour.

References

1. Sicherman B, Green CH. Notable American women: the modern period: a biographical dictionary. Cambridge, MA: The Belknap Press of Harvard University Press; 1980.
2. Damrosch DS. Dorothy Hansine Andersen. J Pediatr. 1964;65:477–9.
3. Tregaskis S. Women—long denied a role at P&S—helped shape medicine in the 20th century. Columbia Medicine (Spring/Summer), 2016.
4. Dorothy H. Andersen papers. Archives at the Augustus C. Long Health Sciences Library of Columbia University.
5. Andersen DH. Lymphatics of the fallopian tube of the sow/by Dorothy H. Andersen, Contributions to embryology, vol. 19, no. 102. Washington, DC: Carnegie Institution of Washington; 1927.
6. Andersen DH. The rate of passage of the mammalian ovum through various portions of the fallopian tube. Am J Physiol. 1927;82(3):557–69.
7. Andersen DH. Lymphatics of the fallopian tube of the sow/by Dorothy H. Andersen, Contributions to embryology; vol. 19, no. 102. Washington, DC: Carnegie Institution of Washington; 1927.
8. Corner GW. Hormones in human reproduction. Princeton University Press; 1942.
9. Machol L. Ahead of her time: a biography of Dorothy H. Andersen, M.D.
10. Corner GW. George Linius Streeter 1873–1948, a biographical memoir. National Academy Biographical memoirs, vol. 28. Washington, DC: National Academy of Science; 1954. p. 261–87.

A Reboot

5

In the summer of 1929, Dorothy Andersen started work as an assistant in pathology at Presbyterian Hospital in CUMC; she would be linked to Columbia University's Department of Pathology for the rest of her life.

Construction of CUMC began in 1925 and continued for several years over contiguous blocks in northwest Manhattan's Washington Heights neighborhood. This new medical center would eventually include a general hospital for adults (Presbyterian Hospital) and another for children (Babies Hospital), several more specialty hospitals (including one for neurology patients, another for obstetric and gynecology patients, and another for psychiatry patients), as well as outpatient clinics and several allied health schools and colleges of Columbia University. However at CUMC's opening in 1928, it included only the Presbyterian Hospital, the Sloane Hospital for Women (a hospital dedicated to obstetrics and gynecology), the Vanderbilt Clinic, and Columbia University's College of Physicians and Surgeons (the university's medical school). In 1929 both the Neurologic Institute and Babies Hospital were added: Babies Hospital moved from its former location on the east side of Manhattan into its new CUMC location later that same year just a few months shy of the Great Depression. In spite of the economic disruption associated with the Great Depression, CUMC was about to become one of the largest medical centers in the United States.

Andersen was still a young woman when she began her pathology career: she was not a fan of personal photos, and she always maintained a self-deprecatory attitude regarding her appearance. As a result, photos of her in the 1930s are mostly unavailable, so one is left to speculate about her appearance based on the few available photos of her younger and older self: she was about five feet four or five inches tall and of average weight – though a bit stockier when she entered middle age. She had a somewhat casual approach to dress and grooming but was certainly not disheveled. Her hair was cut shorter than it had been as a student. Though she may have been a smoker early in her career [1], she was not described as a "chain smoker" until the 1950s [2]. Her voice (from a professional recording in the late

J. S. Baird, *Dorothy Hansine Andersen*,
https://doi.org/10.1007/978-3-030-87484-1_5

1950s) was soft and musical. In July 1929 as she began her career in pathology, her appearance was non-threatening, unpretentious, and a bit informal.

Her living arrangements were also unpretentious and a bit informal: her mailing address in the mid-1930s was Bard Hall, a Columbia University dormitory adjacent to CUMC. It opened its doors in 1931, and it is possible Andersen was an early resident. It was convenient and inexpensive, and she would have been happy to be there, as it offered an opportunity to save some money. While there were few luxuries available, many of the dormitory rooms had beautiful views of the Hudson River and the George Washington Bridge (also opened in 1931), as subsequent generations of medical students at Columbia University's College of Physicians and Surgeons can attest.[1]

The choice of pathology was a good choice for her to make, as it provided her with some flexibility in a future career which would lean heavily on her earlier training in anatomy and surgery. However, it is not known why she chose Columbia University as her new academic home: she had no strong personal ties to the city and no known academic ties to Columbia University. One can only guess about her motivation; it is possible that Beryl Paige (who graduated from Mount Holyoke in 1911 and in 1928 was a resident physician in pathology at CUMC) or Florence Sabin (then at the Rockefeller Institute on Manhattan's east side) influenced her choice. It is likely just coincidental that another Mount Holyoke graduate – Virginia Apgar[2] – entered medical school at Columbia University's College of Physicians and Surgeons in 1929. Perhaps Andersen was aware and excited by the rapid growth and development of this new medical center in New York City. As much of her childhood was spent in an area of New Jersey adjacent to Manhattan (where her father worked), it is also possible that she was attracted to the hustle and bustle of the big city: she certainly enjoyed the city's many cultural attractions, including theatrical and musical events [3, 4].

It is interesting to speculate from almost a century later that pathology in the 1930s may have offered much the same allure as anatomy did to an earlier generation of physicians in the first decade of the twentieth century: both pursuits mandated extensive time in a laboratory, as well as expertise with a variety of technologies, and answers to clinical questions delivered by renowned practitioners of either pursuit were generally accepted as definitive.[3] Pathologists might have had the ability to set their own agenda for research in the 1930s: if you did chance upon an interesting clinical finding as a pathologist, it was up to you to determine the means and manner of investigation at your own laboratory bench; such investigations might be less feasible in a strictly clinical practice (i.e., pediatrics or internal medicine), as there might not be an available laboratory bench. As Andersen noted years later: "it (pathology) enables the physician to keep one foot in the wards,

---

[1] Including the author of this biography.

[2] Apgar graduated from Mount Holyoke College three years after Andersen.

[3] The Department of Anatomy and Cell Biology at Columbia University eventually merged with the Department of Pathology (to form the Department of Pathology and Cell Biology) in the late 1980s, affirming some of the common aims of anatomists and pathologists.

where medical problems exist, and the other in the laboratory, where facilities for solving the problems are available" [4]. While certainly true for Dorothy Andersen, not all pathologists were able to keep one foot in the wards.

With the identification of specific bacteria associated with a specific disease, and the subsequent recognition that certain antibiotics killed bacteria at the same time that they also cured disease, the germ theory became well-accepted in academic medicine in the early twentieth century. As a result, pathologists assumed more responsibility for identifying patients with an infectious disease. For example, meningitis was often diagnosed by a pathologist (e.g., Martha Wollstein at Babies Hospital) who noted the presence of specific bacteria with inflammatory cells in the fluid around the brain (the cerebrospinal fluid), whether that fluid was examined before (i.e., from a lumbar puncture during life[4]) or after death (i.e., at autopsy). Pathologists became essential members of the medical team, a development which may also have influenced Andersen's career choice.

To help frame her career choice, it is important to consider the definition, associated procedures, and context of an autopsy examination. An autopsy is a surgical procedure performed by a pathologist on a human corpse in order to identify the cause(s) of death and disease. Standardization of autopsy procedures and testing began in the nineteenth century and continued with advances in biomedical technology throughout the twentieth century. An autopsy was already a complex procedure in 1929, and many academic pathologists, like Wollstein, worked at the cutting edge of medical science. Though perhaps a bit less important currently with the development of less invasive diagnostic techniques, autopsies continue to have considerable forensic importance [5].

Andersen learned quickly what was expected of her as a pathologist: her expertise as an anatomist and her surgical training gave her a head start. Autopsy records reveal that she performed autopsies on her own in the summer of 1929 at Presbyterian Hospital. Paige was then the Assistant Pathologist at Babies Hospital and performed autopsies primarily at Babies Hospital and at Sloane Hospital for Women (on stillborn babies or neonates who died), but also occasionally at Presbyterian Hospital. It is possible that Paige also offered advice and mentorship to Andersen.

Though there is no indication they were close friends, their backgrounds suggest shared experiences and interests: like Andersen, Paige was an only child and a Mount Holyoke graduate with a deep and abiding commitment to research. In addition, Paige had what might seem to be a false start, as well as a profound interest in higher education: she taught zoology at Mount Holyoke College prior to graduating with an M.A. from Columbia University in 1917 (so Paige's tenure at Mount Holyoke ended before Andersen's undergraduate career began), and Paige then worked as a bacteriologist before graduating from Columbia University's College of Physicians and Surgeons with an M.D. in 1924.[5]

---

[4] In 1911 Wollstein wrote about the emerging utility of lumbar punctures: "The extension of the practice of employing lumbar puncture as an aid to the diagnosis of meningitis has had, as one effect, the establishment of the important fact that the influenza bacillus [i.e., Hemophilus influenzae] is a not infrequent cause of seropurulent meningitis."

[5] This was only the fourth class of medical students at Columbia University to include women.

Autopsy records of Presbyterian Hospital from 1929 through 1935 reveal the variety of pathologic findings in almost every adult patient examined by Andersen or Paige and the need for them to exercise the detective skills of a Sherlock Holmes. Acutely ill adults often had several occult and chronic diseases in addition to whatever was responsible for their acute illness. Determining the underlying cause of death was often tricky:

- A 28-year-old female who died with clinical diagnoses of acute rheumatic fever, chronic kidney disease, and streptococcal bacteremia[6] was examined by Andersen. She noted dark brown granular pigment in the spleen and granulomas in mediastinal lymph nodes – indicating a history of malaria (still endemic in some parts of New York City prior to mosquito abatement efforts in the early twentieth century), as well as tuberculosis. Also present was a diseased heart valve – the mitral valve was inflamed and thickened, and bacterial vegetations were present – indicating a history of rheumatic fever with resultant mitral valve stenosis and eventually acute bacterial endocarditis.[7] Andersen also noted acute glomerulonephritis[8] and an infected uterine stump associated with a hysterectomy 4 years previously. As Andersen noted, "The case is interesting but complicated": she suggested that an earlier episode of rheumatic fever damaged the mitral valve and chronic infection of the uterine stump with *Streptococcus* (likely *Streptococcus pyogenes*, though identification of this species was not yet routinely available) led to acute bacterial endocarditis and acute glomerulonephritis. This was a very astute guess on Andersen's part, as we now know that *Streptococcus pyogenes* is associated with both the development of rheumatic fever and a type of glomerulonephritis, thus tying several of these diagnoses together (though not, of course, the history of malaria or tuberculosis).
- A 57-year-old man died with a pulmonary hemorrhage and a history of emphysema. At an autopsy examination by Paige, she noted an acute aortic aneurysm which catastrophically ruptured into his trachea and lungs. She discovered the aneurysm was due to late syphilis involving the aorta, with additional involvement of the aortic valve (in the heart) and fibrosis of heart muscle.

At the same time that Andersen was learning how to be a pathologist, she was also beginning to work on another advanced degree to complete the research she began at Hopkins as a medical student: a degree of Doctor of Medical Sciences (Med.Sc.D.)[9] at Columbia University. Nearly a decade's worth of work – with over a dozen related publications – culminated in her dissertation in 1935: "The relation of the endocrine glands to the female reproductive cycle." Her dissertation appeared around the same time that some understanding of female ovulation and pregnancy

---

[6] The presence of bacteria in the bloodstream, an indication that the infection is severe.

[7] A bacterial infection of the heart.

[8] An inflammatory disease of the kidneys.

[9] A Med.Sc.D. degree in the first half of the twentieth century was a doctorate degree (i.e., similar to a Ph.D.).

was accumulating dramatically: the actions of estrogen (Andersen knew this as "ovarian hormone" in the 1930's) had been described in the early 1920s, but it was not isolated until 1929, while the discovery of progesterone (another ovarian hormone) occurred in 1930 in George Corner's laboratory at the University of Rochester (Andersen's mentor from 1926 to 1927). In addition, luteinizing hormone and follicle-stimulating hormone – both from the anterior pituitary – were discovered in 1931, but their roles in the female reproductive cycle were still being worked out at the time of Andersen's dissertation, while the discovery of gonadotropin-releasing hormone from the hypothalamus lay several decades in the future. Andersen would surely have been aware of the rapid pace of these discoveries during the 1930s, including Corner's role, and the impact of these discoveries on her own work.

The decade of the 1930s was an exciting time for academic researchers specializing in female reproduction, but at some point Andersen realized that it was still a bit early to offer an overview of the mammalian female reproductive system: even a meticulous anatomist could not hope to solve the complex interplay of the pituitary and ovarian hormones during the estrus cycle just by looking at slides, however prettily stained, from a number of different organs and species. Nevertheless, she was able to offer some context to the relationship between the organs responsible for female reproduction and the other endocrine organs:

> The hypothesis as to the regulation of the oestrus cycle which best fits the evidence at present known is that of a cyclic reciprocal stimulation of the ovary and the hypophysis. The alterations in the thyroid, liver and adrenal occurring during the female reproductive cycle are secondary to those in the hypophysis and ovary.

She was awarded a doctorate degree in June 1935. With only a few minor exceptions [6, 7], Andersen left this chapter of her academic life entirely behind when Martha Wollstein retired that same year: Beryl Paige took Wollstein's position as Babies Hospital's Pathologist, and in July 1935 Andersen took over as Babies Hospital's Assistant Pathologist.

Andersen continued to work at Babies Hospital for the rest of her life.

References

1. Ores C. Interview with Celia Ores, J.S. Baird, Editor. 2021.
2. Doershuk CF. Cystic fibrosis in the 20th century: people, events, and progress. Cleveland: AM Publishing Ltd; 2001.
3. Machol L. Ahead of her time: a biography of Dorothy H. Andersen, M.D.
4. Dorothy H. Andersen papers. Archives at the Augustus C. Long Health Sciences Library of Columbia University.
5. Clark MJ. Autopsy. Lancet. 2005;366(9499):1767.
6. Victor J, Andersen DH. Stimulation of anterior hypophysis metabolism by theelin or dihydrotheelin. Am J Physiol. 1937;120(1):154–66.
7. Andersen DH, Sperry WM. A study of cholesterol in the adrenal gland in different phases of reproduction in the female rat. J Physiol. 1937;90(3):296–302.

Part II

Babies Hospital During the McIntosh Era

In accumulating property for ourselves or our posterity, in founding a family or a state, or acquiring fame even, we are mortal; but in dealing with truth we are immortal, and need fear no change or accident.

Henry David Thoreau: On Walden Pond

Babies Hospital in New York City was one of the first hospitals in the United States dedicated to the care of the very young when it was founded in the late nineteenth century. In 1929 it joined Columbia University at the site of a new medical center in Manhattan, and since then Babies Hospital has served as the focal point of the university's Department of Pediatrics. The McIntosh Era from 1931 to 1960 at Babies Hospital was the setting for Andersen's career: the Chair of Pediatrics at Columbia University's College of Physicians and Surgeons and the medical director at Babies Hospital over these three decades was Rustin McIntosh. He was the heir of L. Emmett Holt, Sr; both were critical to the early development of pediatrics in the United States. McIntosh also played a major role in support of Andersen's career, including recognition of her skills as a clinician, though their relationship may have been a bit distant. Andersen's personality and inclinations were much less conservative than McIntosh's; nevertheless, each was aware and respectful of the other's value and skill.

Babies Hospital's first pathologist was Martha Wollstein: she began training at Babies Hospital shortly after Holt was appointed medical director, and the end of her career overlapped the first few years of the McIntosh Era. Her accomplishments went mostly unappreciated for several decades after she retired, though nearly a century later it is clear that she was "the first fully specialized pediatric perinatal pathologist practicing exclusively in a North America children's hospital, [and] she also blazed another pathway as a very early pioneer female clinician-scientist [38]." Wollstein's career served in some respects as another model for Andersen, who joined Babies Hospital as Assistant Pathologist upon Wollstein's retirement, and quickly began to study a new disease characterized by cysts and fibrosis in the pancreas of young children.

During the decade following her landmark 1938 study of CF, Andersen developed important diagnostic and treatment strategies for this new disease. She spent the remainder of her career actively engaged in a variety of clinical pursuits and research, both in pathology as well as in pediatrics, all the while maintaining a separate focus on CF. Attempts to minimize Andersen's contributions to the care of CF suggest gender bias and the Matilda Effect (a bias against acknowledging the achievements of women scientists by attributing their achievements to men).

Many of the Babies Hospital faculty during the McIntosh Era achieved academic renown. Brief sketches of some of Andersen's colleagues, as well as historical notes regarding Babies Hospital, provide a context for Andersen's career. Synergy played a role in some of the accomplishments of Andersen and her colleagues. While Andersen would have been successful wherever she worked, it is remarkable how many of her female colleagues—including Hattie Alexander, Virginia Apgar, and Hilde Bruch—enjoyed careers at the highest levels of academic medicine.

Andersen's medical expertise, honesty, and sympathetic nature ensured that her patients and their families loved her. A valentine sent by one of her patients also suggested a painful truth about medical care for patients with CF during the first few decades following her landmark study in 1938: "To Dr. Andersen who has pulled me through many a tough year." Living with CF in the twentieth century was a constant battle, in spite of therapeutic advances: survival was never assured, and medical progress incremental.

Andersen was a vital participant in that battle.

Historical Perspectives

Hospitals for infants and children emerged in Europe during the first half of the nineteenth century, but it wasn't till the second half of the century that they began to appear in the United States. Babies Hospital in New York City was founded in June 1887 by five women: Sarah and Julia McNutt, Jeannie Smith, Isabella Satterthwaite, and Isabella Banks; the McNutt sisters were the first attending physicians at Babies Hospital.[1]

A city-wide survey several years earlier by Sarah McNutt noted only 10 hospital beds dedicated to young children (out of 10,000 total hospital beds) [1] during a time when infant mortality was much higher than currently,[2] so a hospital for young children must have seemed like low-hanging fruit to physicians anxious to improve the health of children. The implications of McNutt's observations now seem obvious: some infants and children who get sick and need medical care should be treated in the hospital, like sick adults. However, the knowledge needed to provide better hospital care and improved outcomes for sick infants and children was slow to develop.

Infectious diseases were responsible for most infant deaths, and improved public health was a necessary first step for any realistic plan to decrease infant or childhood mortality. In the late eighteenth century, an outbreak of yellow fever led to the creation of the New York City Board of Health, and quarantines were commonly ordered for yellow fever and cholera epidemics in the nineteenth century. Rapid metropolitan growth meant it was the largest and most congested metropolis in the United States, and the poorest residents lived in the most congested areas. Pigs

---

[1] It was not, strictly speaking, the first hospital established for the care of children in New York City: in 1857 the New York Infirmary for Indigent Women and Children was established by Elizabeth Blackwell.

[2] The infant mortality rate (a ratio of the number of infants that die annually compared to those that are born during the same time period) in the United States during the first few years of the twentieth century was at least 100/1000 live births; by the end of the century it had dropped to 7/1000 live births.

J. S. Baird, *Dorothy Hansine Andersen*,
https://doi.org/10.1007/978-3-030-87484-1_6

commonly roamed the streets of Manhattan until the middle of the nineteenth century – and represented a valuable financial asset for many of the city's poor – though their presence also contributed to public health problems. Sewage and water supply problems were worse in the poorest Manhattan neighborhoods and were often associated with outbreaks of cholera and typhus [2]. Outbreaks of smallpox, influenza, and typhoid fever were also common at the end of the nineteenth century in New York City. As a first step, sewage control and the security of the water supply were important public health goals by the late nineteenth century. Hospitals dedicated to the care of sick infants and children were not far behind.

There were, however, obstacles to the development of Babies Hospital: a neighbor objected to the first hospital site (and suggested that infectious diseases would threaten the neighborhood), and an injunction prevented operations there (at 45th and Lexington Avenue) leading to a 5,000 dollar loss when it was sold. Another temporary site was suitable for only a year or so. It was not until 1889 that a brownstone on Manhattan's east side (at 55th St. and Lexington Avenue) was purchased and developed as a more permanent hospital site: eventually it housed 8 wards with 68 beds for children up to the age of 3 years. Sarah McNutt wrote that "The medical work, however, grew so rapidly, and encroached so much upon our private work, that we felt obliged to withdraw from the Babies' Hospital a year after assisting in founding it" [3]. Unfortunately, gender bias was not uncommon in this era, and whether that also contributed to their withdrawal is unknown, though it would not be surprising. Financial support of this new entity was, apparently, then precarious, and it was not until Luther Emmett Holt, Sr. was hired as medical director in 1889 that significant financial backing was obtained and the debt and finances successfully reorganized [4]. Whether Holt's selection represented another example of gender bias would also not be surprising.

Luther Emmett Holt, Sr.

The last decade of the nineteenth century was notable for the publication of two textbooks which helped inform and modernize their respective fields of medicine. William Osler, often referred to as "The Father of Modern Medicine," wrote "The Principles and Practice of Medicine" (published in 1892) and forever changed the practice of internal (adult) medicine. Several years after joining Babies Hospital as its medical director, Holt finished work on his "Diseases of Infancy and Childhood," and it was accepted for publication in 1897 and published in 1898:

> Holt's book … in simple clear language, was at once recognized in this country as the standard text on pediatrics, occupying a place corresponding to Osler's textbook on internal medicine. All medical students were given it to study and it was the pediatric reference book for all practitioners. During Holt's lifetime, in successively revised forms, it ran through eleven editions and was translated into Chinese! [5]

Holt was later referred to as the "Osler of Pediatrics" [2]. His textbook has been revised numerous times since his death; it also changed – and helped define – the practice of pediatrics. Both textbooks (Osler's and Holt's) categorized diseases by organ system and included whatever scientific information was available for each disease (Fig. 6.1).

Along with keeping up to date with the emerging medical literature, both authors regarded clinical experience with patients as essential for medical students. They also believed that the study of pathology – including in particular microscopy and other laboratory tools used to study a disease process on a cellular (or smaller) level – were essential to medical advances.

Holt graduated with an M.D. from Columbia University's College of Physicians and Surgeons in 1880 and then completed an internship in surgery at Bellevue Hospital (where William Welch was also beginning his career; Welch would later become the first dean of Johns Hopkins School of Medicine). For several years Holt pursued a private practice in pediatrics and was affiliated with several hospitals in the New York City area.

Holt joined Babies Hospital in 1889 and gradually became a leader in the growing specialty of pediatrics, eventually becoming "the leading pediatrician of the day" [6]. In 1897 Holt was named the President of the American Pediatric Society; he accumulated numerous related international responsibilities over the next few decades. He was renowned both as a teacher and as a master clinician, and he was connected socially to some of the city's elite: "he knew John D. Rockefeller and was instrumental in persuading him to endow the Rockefeller Institute for Medical Research and together with William Welch was one of the original members of the Board of Scientific Directors" [6].

Though his character and personality reflect his era in ways that may seem a bit unusual over a century later, Holt provided a model for others to follow (in particular for Rustin McIntosh, one of Holt's interns, who later assumed Holt's position at Babies Hospital):

> Holt was a small man; his voice was quiet and clear and his movements alert and quick. Always immaculately dressed, he rarely smiled or laughed and appeared to be driven by a stern sense of duty. Hard working, efficient, thorough and meticulous in his work, he also possessed sound judgment, intellectual honesty, and a total dedication to the welfare of his patients. Children were treated as individuals. He remarked that "the best way to make friends with a child is not to try". He was not interested in speculation, nor was he possessed of an imaginative mind. His approach was always intensely practical and concerned with knowledge that might help to solve problems. Besides being a great clinician, he was also a born teacher. His interests extended beyond the illnesses of children to a wish to ensure that they grew up healthy—physically, mentally, and morally. In this he was decades ahead of most of his contemporaries throughout the world. Holt developed fixed routines in management which were applied with vigour. He expected the highest standards from his assistants but never gave praise or formed close friendships. Nor was he ever unkind. [4]

Though he rarely smiled or laughed, and some felt he lacked a sense of humor [6], it is probably more accurate to say that he had a very dry sense of humor:

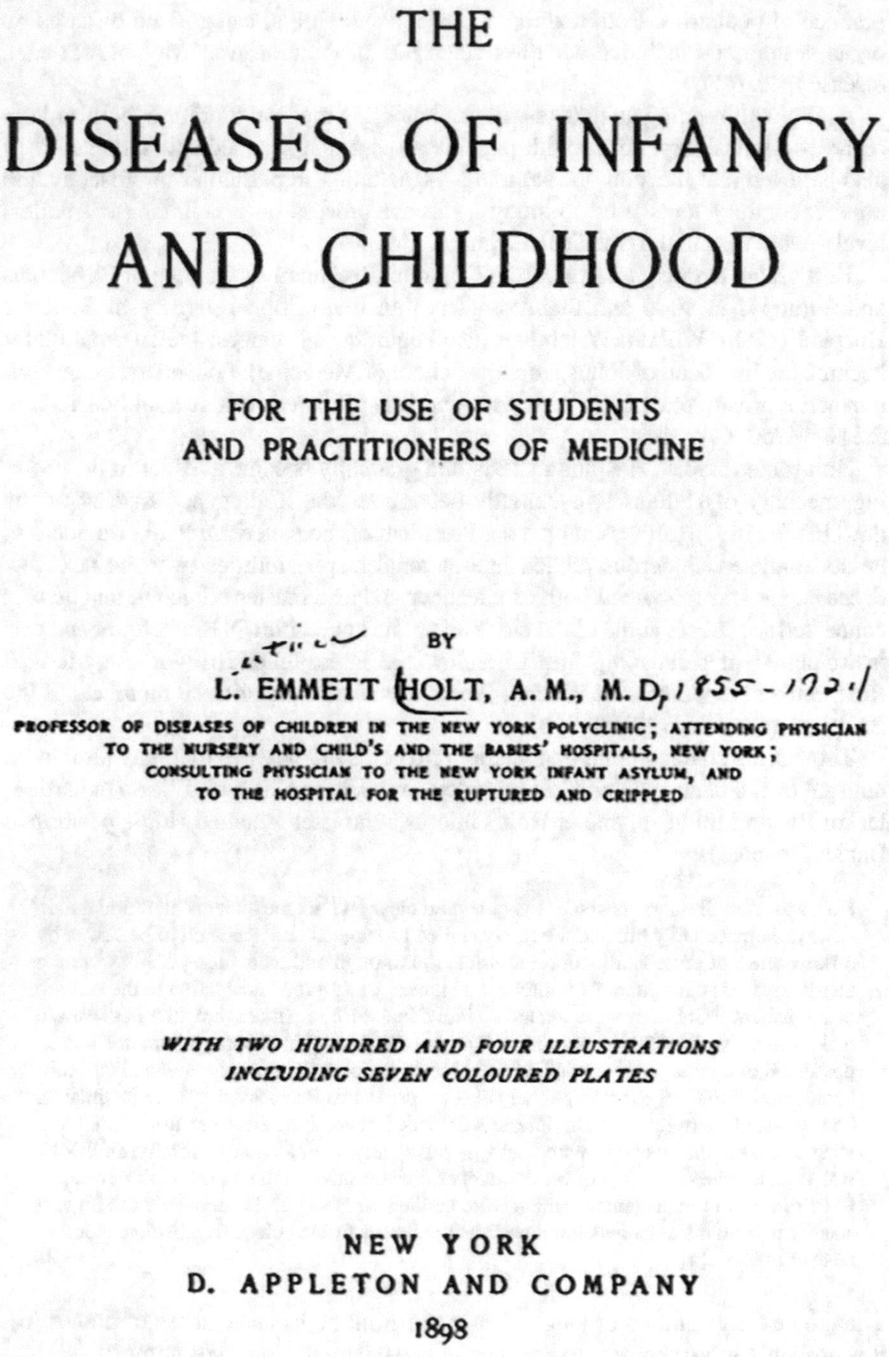

THE

DISEASES OF INFANCY

AND CHILDHOOD

FOR THE USE OF STUDENTS
AND PRACTITIONERS OF MEDICINE

BY

L. EMMETT HOLT, A. M., M. D, *1855 - 1721*

PROFESSOR OF DISEASES OF CHILDREN IN THE NEW YORK POLYCLINIC; ATTENDING PHYSICIAN
TO THE NURSERY AND CHILD'S AND THE BABIES' HOSPITALS, NEW YORK;
CONSULTING PHYSICIAN TO THE NEW YORK INFANT ASYLUM, AND
TO THE HOSPITAL FOR THE RUPTURED AND CRIPPLED

*WITH TWO HUNDRED AND FOUR ILLUSTRATIONS
INCLUDING SEVEN COLOURED PLATES*

NEW YORK
D. APPLETON AND COMPANY
1898

Fig. 6.1 Title page of the first edition of Holt's textbook. (In the public domain)

Rustin McIntosh relates that when Dr. Holt had finished examining a child brought in by a young doctor with a diagnosis of appendicitis, he [Holt] observed, "Doctor, the trouble is not with the Appendix; it is with the Table of Contents." [5]

McIntosh reminisced that Holt "had [a] genial humour and a stock of lively anecdotes" [7] (Fig. 6.2).

Babies Hospital became a teaching affiliate of Columbia University's College of Physicians and Surgeons in 1900. In 1901, Holt succeeded Abraham Jacobi as Professor of Pediatrics at the College of Physicians and Surgeons. In 1902 a renovation of Babies Hospital – including an elevator, a telephone, more beds, an X-ray machine, and a solarium – was completed. Babies Hospital then grew even more rapidly, acquiring pediatric specialists with expertise in pathology and surgery. Holt continued to direct activities, though he was frequently called away to deal with issues at other institutions or professional organizations during this period of rapid growth in pediatrics. He is credited with a variety of innovations during his tenure at Babies Hospital, including providing instruction and a textbook for nursing

Fig. 6.2 Luther Emmett Holt, Sr. early in the twentieth century. (Courtesy of the National Library of Medicine)

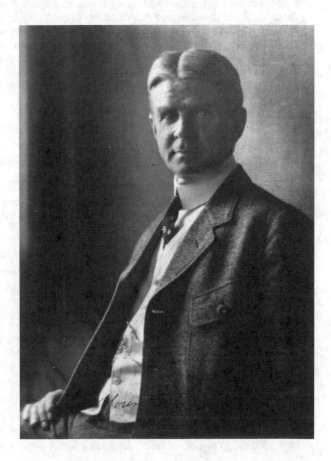

students, advocating the importance of a bedside medical record, and recognizing and recruiting talented physicians.

For the first two decades of the twentieth century, the identity of Babies Hospital was closely linked to Holt, as remembered by McIntosh:

> Dr. Holt for many years *was* Babies Hospital, dominating the selection of the attending staff, appointing the house staff, determining the diagnostic and therapeutic policies including nursing practices and procedures, and in general conducting a benevolent dictatorship... When a dispute arose about the diagnosis in a difficult clinical problem the case would be presented to Dr. Holt at grand rounds, he would make his own examination, announce his diagnosis, and that was that- the final word. [7]

As both social custom and pediatric care began to evolve, Holt's "benevolent dictatorship" seemed to some a bit less benevolent in the decades following his death. William Silverman compared Holt to Holt's successor McIntosh, to McIntosh's benefit in the mid-1940s:

> In the old hospital on Lexington and 55th St, caste distinctions were sharp and immutable. Freddy (Dr. Bartlett) remembered a daily ritual: the hospital elevator was brought down to the main floor at the same time every morning to await the arrival of the chief, L. Emmett Holt, Sr. A porter was posted on Lexington Avenue to spot the great man, he ran and held the door open as Holt swept in, entered the elevator without loss of stride, and was whisked up to the top floor to begin very solemn rounds. The contrast between Freddy's Babies Hospital of memory and the one I found could not have been more extreme. Rusty McIntosh, our chief, had no strutting airs and he had a completely disarming style of leadership- he led by quiet example. [8]

However, it was most likely that same elevator man whose actions suggested that Babies Hospital under Holt might not have been as austere or forbidding as Silverman seemed to suggest. From the Babies Hospital Historical Archives:

> Letter to Miss Smith who was superintendent of the Babies Hospital for many years, from the elevator operator who had been with the hospital for a long time. He was away on a vacation in Atlantic City spending $30 a week for board and lodging but feeling this was worthwhile to 'live the life' for two weeks:

> 'I diagnosed today a case of pyloric stenosis. A couple staying at our cottage from Philadelphia with a nursing baby. The baby has been vomiting after every feeding for two weeks. She had a doctor here and he blamed the mother's milk. She was out on the porch with the baby after nursing it and I saw it shoot out like a fountain. I had her give the baby some boiled water and I showed her the waves which were distinct. I told her to take a trip to New York and see Doctor Downes but she went back to see her family doctor. I told her to tell him that the elevator man from Babies Hospital, New York diagnosed the case as positive Pyloric Stenosis'. [9]

The symptoms and signs reported by the elevator man do indeed suggest pyloric stenosis, and the tone and concern of his observations suggest that the older Babies Hospital was a bit more liberal – at least in educating elevator men – than Silverman's story might suggest (other than close attendance by the elevator man at medical rounds or lectures, how else to explain his expertise?). In any case, the rapid evolution of pediatric care would soon make it difficult for many physicians – not to mention elevator men – to keep up with current medical practice.

In large part, this was due to the rapid pace of the incorporation of science into medical care in the first half of the twentieth century: numerous unhelpful therapies were weeded out and replaced with therapies rooted in a more scientific understanding of disease, and that process continues more than a century later. Richard Day noted in 1987: "Rusty [McIntosh] once asked me to look over a file of Holt's case records. There were 300 charts of patients from all over the world. Many were of medical interest, but none contained a treatment recommendation that would be considered useful today" [10]. Indeed, some of the treatment recommendations from the first edition of Holt's pediatric textbook appear a bit odd:

- "the first step in treatment of acute pharyngitis is to open the bowels freely by means of calomel, castor oil, or magnesia."
- "during the attacks [of stomach pains] the patient should be put to bed, and counter-irritation used over the stomach, best by means of a turpentine stupe or a mustard paste."

Many nursing practices from this early era of pediatrics also appear primitive. It is helpful, however, to remember that many of the therapies used today to treat sick children in the most academically advanced hospitals are likely to appear less than useful 50 to 100 years from now. Before concluding that Holt's expertise as a clinician was negligible by modern standards, consider the comments from two of his students (Howard Mason and Edwards Park), each of whom went on to successful careers in academic medicine:

> How good a practitioner was he? When one considers how he continually tabulated and analyzed his increasingly large experience, the meticulous care with which he studied his patients and the acuteness of his perceptions and psychological intuition, he probably had no equal in this country at the height of his career. In his later years some of the rising generation, trained in the laboratory and in the newer viewpoints, surpassed him in certain fields of child care, but it is doubtful if even they excelled him in the handling of day-after-day problems. [5]

Babies Hospital provided the setting for much of the evolution of pediatric care in the early twentieth century, and Holt had an important role in that evolution. Two of the physicians Holt chose to staff Babies Hospital were critically important in solidifying his legacy as well as the reputation of Babies Hospital: Martha Wollstein and Rustin McIntosh. Holt, Wollstein, and McIntosh were also critically important – for different reasons – to Dorothy Andersen.

Martha Wollstein

A marriage of sorts between the practice of medicine and scientific research followed several related events over a century ago: the founding of both the Johns Hopkins University School of Medicine and the Rockefeller Institute, coupled with the publication of the Flexner report on medical education. Though it might now seem inevitable, a scientific foundation for medical care in the United States only became explicit early in the twentieth century, related at least in part to these three events.

When Johns Hopkins University's School of Medicine opened in 1893, physicians responsible for its philosophy and direction included William Osler and William Welch, both of whom are now recognized as pioneers in the modern practice of medicine. Their medical school became an exemplary center of medical education and research in addition to clinical care. In 1902 the Rockefeller Institute for Medical Research was established in New York City with William Welch as the first President of its Board of Scientific Directors and Simon Flexner (who trained under Welch) as the Institute's first Director. As a biomedical research center, the institute's early goals centered principally on investigations of infectious diseases which had a major impact on public health, and it extended grants to researchers of those diseases. In 1910 the Rockefeller Institute's hospital opened, permitting clinical research to occur on the institute's campus. Also in 1910, the Carnegie Foundation sponsored a broad review of US medical education by Abraham Flexner – Simon's brother. The resulting Flexner report suggested that numerous changes in medical education were needed, "formalizing the Hopkins model of critical, hospital-based teaching" [11]. This model represented the incorporation of scientific evidence with a humanistic approach: clinical experience with real patients in realistic settings was viewed as essential, in ways exemplified particularly by Osler.

However, the Flexner report was not without controversy. The numbers of medical schools and medical students were markedly reduced as a direct result of the report (as schools unable to comply with the requirements of this new model were closed), limiting – at least in theory – the possibility that women or minorities would be able to get a medical education. Over a century later in 2019, women made up – for the first time – a majority of medical students in the United States, but this was nowhere close to the situation in the early twentieth century. Women were only accepted then to a few medical schools, and the number of women medical students in those schools was quite small.

The first woman to earn a medical degree in the United States was Elizabeth Blackwell: she graduated in 1849 from Geneva Medical College (later absorbed into Syracuse University and later still into the State University of New York), and she opened the New York Infirmary for Indigent Women and Children in New York City's Greenwich Village in 1857. A little over a decade later, Elizabeth and her sister Emily Blackwell (also a physician) founded the Women's Medical College of the New York Infirmary. Sarah McNutt (one of the founders of Babies Hospital) was an early graduate from the Women's Medical College of the New York Infirmary in 1877.

Of note, the first class of women medical students at Johns Hopkins University's School of Medicine began their studies with that school's first student class in 1893 (the university was constrained by financial considerations to agree to admit women when it opened), while Columbia University's College of Physicians and Surgeons did not admit women until 1917 and Harvard University Medical School did not admit women until 1945 (as 1917 and 1945 were both concurrent with a world war, the pool of men seeking admission was then much diminished, leading to a more serious consideration of women as medical students).

As a result, the options for medical education in the United States for women in the nineteenth century, as well as the first half of the twentieth century, were limited; in 1889 Martha Wollstein graduated from the Women's Medical College of the New York Infirmary. In 1890 she began her medical training at Babies Hospital as its first intern. After completing her training in 1891, she was hired as Babies Hospital's first pathologist [12], though she likely had numerous other hospital duties. She developed an interest in infectious diseases, particularly bacteriology. In 1896 a pathology laboratory was added to Babies Hospital, and Wollstein's research efforts were then more focused. At the beginning of the twentieth century, Babies Hospital became affiliated with Columbia University and entered a phase of rapid growth, including both the facility and its medical staff. Among those hired by Holt was Dorothy Reed as a resident physician in 1903; she was recommended to Holt by William Welch.

Dorothy Reed's background was quite different from Wollstein's: Reed and Florence Sabin (Dorothy Andersen's mentor) were classmates[3] and friends at the Johns Hopkins University School of Medicine. Both were recognized as honors graduates and entitled to choose their internships, and both chose internal medicine under the direction of William Osler [6]. Reed continued to work for a few years at Hopkins following her internship, mostly in pathology; she identified the Reed-Sternberg cell (associated with Hodgkin's disease). She remained friendly with Osler and often stayed with his family when she visited Baltimore [6].

While at Babies Hospital, Reed became friendly with Wollstein, though it appears that neither Reed nor Wollstein developed much of a friendship with Holt [6]: Holt's stern demeanor and devotion to duty certainly did not encourage friendship. Moreover, friendships between married men and young, single women were actively discouraged. Like Osler, Holt favored clinical activities over laboratory work and took advantage of Reed's expertise in pathology to get her help interpreting pathology specimens for his studies [6]. Wollstein informed Reed that Holt no longer asked for her assistance in that context, as she was in the habit of billing Holt for this extracurricular service. When Reed did the same, Holt apparently paid her once but did not ask her for further assistance [6].

Reed's patience with Holt began to evaporate, particularly as she began to learn about the economics of academic medicine in New York City compared to what she had experienced in Baltimore. She suggested to Holt that "in six years in Baltimore I never heard money mentioned in regard to the practice of medicine [6]", though it was a frequent topic at Babies Hospital. To be fair to Holt, the financial situation at Babies Hospital was always tenuous: Holt's leadership was apparently crucial to Babies Hospital's survival in its first few years, while the hospital's renovation efforts in 1902 required the first of many significant capital investments.

Reed eventually realized that she could, to some degree, manipulate Holt: "Dorothy soon found that he [Holt] would accept any suggestion of hers couched in

---

[3] In the class of 1900.

terms that intimated that it was what Osler would do at Hopkins" [6]. Wollstein, on the other hand, was not a Hopkins graduate and had no connections with Osler or Welch or any of the other contemporary leaders in academic medicine (except Holt); whatever academic expertise she acquired following her residency at Babies Hospital was hard-won and mostly self-taught.

It is ironic that by the time Reed was a resident physician at Babies Hospital, she was no longer interested in a career in academic medicine, while Wollstein was just beginning hers. In 1903, Wollstein was one of the first researchers to isolate *Shigella*:[4]

> The bacillus Dr. Wollstein had discovered had been isolated by the distinguished patholo-gist Simon Flexner several years before, while studying dysentery in the Philippines; her study attracted his attention, and in 1904 an expanded version was published as a special monograph of the Rockefeller Institute, of which Flexner was the director. Two years later she joined the institute's staff as an assistant, while continuing her work at the Babies Hospital. [13]

Wollstein, like Sabin, eventually excelled in academic medicine by a remarkable devotion to work and a superior intellect, though her medical education and training was not nearly as rigorous or as extensive as Sabin's. Reed left Babies Hospital in 1905 to marry and start a family and did not resume her medical career for several years [6]; difficulties inherent in a career in medicine for a woman in the first decade of the twentieth century did indeed leave little time for a family. Academic medi-cine – in which physicians also pursue scholarly activities with the goal of improv-ing medical care generally – was even more difficult for women to pursue a century ago.

Wollstein's career at the Rockefeller Institute spanned more than a decade (from 1907 until 1921): early during her affiliation with the Institute, Simon Flexner taught her some of the newer laboratory techniques in bacteriology [12], and she collaborated with several renowned researchers[5] before eventually developing her own areas of expertise. Important results from her work at the Institute include: antiserum[6] against meningococcus was easily produced in horses and might have therapeutic utility in infected humans, monkeys may transmit polio virus to each other, both chemical and infectious pneumonia lead to similar defense and repair mechanisms in the lungs, *Haemophilus influenzae* is responsible for many cases of bacterial meningitis in children (and goat antiserum was at least a partially effective treatment in a simian model of this disease), and mumps is transmitted by a virus.

In spite of her successful research career at the Institute, by 1918 Simon Flexner realized that Wollstein was frustrated with her academic rank, and he offered her some support, likely to encourage her to remain: he hired a recent graduate from Columbia University (Rebecca Lancefield) to be her technician [14]. Wollstein

---

[4] A bacteria occasionally responsible for diarrhea.

[5] She collaborated with Harold Amoss on bacterial meningitis, Simon Flexner on polio, and Samuel Meltzer on pneumonia.

[6] Serum from blood which contains specific antibodies.

remained unappeased and eventually left the Institute when she was refused membership:

> Martha Wollstein never achieved membership in the Rockefeller Institute. This, however, is no indication of her merit as an investigator. Though it was relatively easy for a woman to be appointed to the institute during its early years, few advanced very far in rank; the only woman to achieve full membership during the first fifty years of the institute's existence was Florence Sabin. [13]

Membership at the Rockefeller Institute was equivalent to the rank of university professor, and when Sabin joined the Institute in 1925 as a member, she had already been recognized at Hopkins several years earlier as the university's first woman professor; her rank at the Institute was commensurate with her rank at Hopkins.

It has been suggested that Wollstein was as productive as "some of her male colleagues [12]" at the Institute and that "institutional discrimination [12]" on the basis of gender [15] was responsible for her lack of advancement. In spite of her many accomplishments, Wollstein never advanced to the rank of professor at Columbia University either. Ironically, Lancefield was eventually awarded membership at the Institute in 1958.[7]

Another factor which perhaps contributed to Wollstein's departure from the Rockefeller Institute was suggested by Rustin McIntosh decades later: "Dr. Holt, Sr., took her away from the Rockefeller Institute and put her in charge of the B.H. path lab" [7]. This is a bit difficult to reconcile with Wollstein's evident determination to pursue a research career at the Institute: it seems unlikely that she would have given it up at someone else's request, no matter who made the request. However, it is possible that by 1921 Holt was better able to recognize Wollstein's academic expertise and saw real benefit in having Babies Hospital be her sole career focus;[8] by then, Wollstein also realized that she was unlikely ever to be awarded membership and was ready to give up her association with the Institute.

By the summer of 1918, the Spanish flu epidemic helped draw Wollstein's attention away from any conflicts she might have had with the Institute, as she was by then one of the world's experts on *Haemophilus influenzae* (formerly known as Pfeiffer's bacillus): for over a decade after the epidemic, this bacteria was mistakenly assumed to be the underlying cause of Spanish flu. Wollstein questioned the possibility that *Haemophilus influenzae* was responsible [16]:

> The patients' serological reactions indicate the parasitic nature of the bacillus but are not sufficiently stable and clean-cut to signify that Pfeiffer's bacillus is the specific inciting agent of epidemic influenza. They do, however, indicate that the bacillus of Pfeiffer is at least a very common secondary invader in influenza, and that its presence influences the course of the pathological process. [16]

---

[7] In part due to her work with Oswald Avery and Alphonse Dochez to help classify the various species of *Streptococcus* (the Lancefield grouping system).

[8] It is still difficult to understand why Holt—or McIntosh—did not act to promote Wollstein to university professor.

It took over a decade to recognize that Wollstein's suspicions were correct. Influenza viruses were not actually identified until 1933, and the major role of that virus—and not *Haemophilus influenzae*—in the Spanish flu epidemic was not fully realized for several more years.

Beginning in 1921 after she left the Rockefeller Institute, Wollstein "devoted herself to pediatric pathology at Babies Hospital" [13]; her research explored anemia, tuberculosis, and tumors in children, in addition to some of the infectious diseases she had previously studied. She recognized some of the pieces of the clinical puzzles suggested by several types of hemolytic anemias, but laboratory techniques to help answer many of these questions were not yet available. Her studies of tuberculosis in children suggested that it was quite common in New York City children (in 4–5% of all children admitted to Babies Hospital [17] and in 13–14% of all Babies Hospital autopsies [18] early in the twentieth century) and that acquisition of the infection was mostly via the respiratory tract [17]. A small series of children with brain tumors at Babies Hospital suggested to her that posterior fossa tumors with resultant hydrocephalus might be the most frequent presentation of brain tumors in children [19], another astute observation (Fig. 6.3).

Fig. 6.3 Martha Wollstein late in her career at Babies Hospital. (In the public domain)

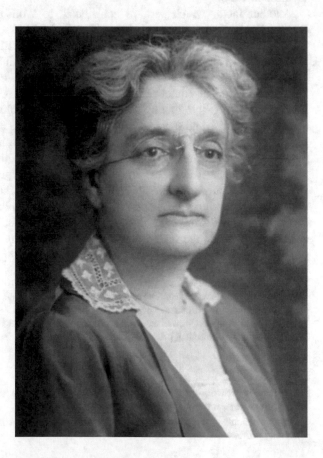

Rustin McIntosh was the Chair of Pediatrics at Babies Hospital for the last few years of Wollstein's career, and he recognized Wollstein's expertise: "She probably had had a more extensive experience in the morphology of disease in infants and children than any other American living" [20]. However he didn't always get along well with her and complained that "we used to fight over details of laboratory procedure" [7]. Wollstein's insight and experience with laboratory procedure both at the Rockefeller Institute and at Babies Hospital suggest that McIntosh would have been unlikely to win those arguments.[9]

Wollstein was described by Dorothy Reed's biographer as:

A rather timid, unassertive woman.... single, very bright, and extremely hardworking but embittered by years of discrimination from the male members of the profession, accentuated in her case by an Orthodox Jewish heritage. [6]

It is true that Wollstein – like Andersen and many of her colleagues at Babies Hospital during the McIntosh Era, including Hattie Alexander, Hilde Bruch, and Virginia Apgar – never married, except to their work. This was also the case for Florence Sabin, the Blackwell sisters, the McNutt sisters, and numerous others. In Wollstein's case, she came from a very supportive and prosperous Manhattan family [15], lived with her parents until their deaths, and was co-executor of her father's estate: at least she did not suffer financial hardship.

However, the above description of Wollstein still seems to miss the mark: she may not have had a forceful, aggressive nature, but she was assertive about her own career and was unlikely to accept the opinion of anyone just because of their academic rank. After all, she left the Rockefeller Institute, never to return. She may have been dissatisfied about certain aspects of her career, but her accomplishments in academic medicine were on the most advanced, cutting edge of science and are inconsistent with a disposition consumed with bitterness. A better understanding of Wollstein's career emerged in this century, long after her death: "Martha Wollstein was not only the first fully specialized pediatric perinatal pathologist practicing exclusively in a North America children's hospital, she also blazed another pathway as a very early pioneer female clinician-scientist" [15]. Wollstein's personality and her academic accomplishments were perhaps difficult to reconcile in an era which was only beginning to appreciate professional women, but it is much easier to recognize the scope of her accomplishments a century later.

An interesting judgment on Wollstein's place in academic pediatrics was made by "RM" after her death: "Of a modest, retiring disposition, she avoided public demonstrations and speechmaking as far as possible; but with those who sought her help as man to man she eagerly shared her wide store of knowledge with open generosity" [20]. This seems a bit more accurate, except for the "man to man" comment. It is very likely that "RM" was Rustin McIntosh, and this was his way of recognizing and lauding Wollstein's accomplishments in a world – and in particular the world of academic pediatrics – dominated by men. Far from being bitter,

---

[9] It is also possible that he had similar disagreements with Andersen, with similar outcomes.

Wollstein was eager to share her knowledge; and while she may have appeared modest and avoided public speeches, she was actually generous as well as successful. She retired in 1935.

By then, Babies Hospital under McIntosh's direction had acquired an important international identity and was a unique institution in New York City; it was a part of one of the largest academic medical centers (CUMC) and associated with one of the oldest medical schools in the United States (Columbia University's College of Physicians and Surgeons). There were 152 beds in Babies Hospital in 1934, including 15 private rooms, over 6 floors [7]. The hospital was also popular among its trainees: William Silverman noted: "All mail came addressed to *The* Babies Hospital, 3975 Broadway (the definite article was an important part of the formal title)." Babies Hospital retained an independent corporate identity until it was completely merged into Presbyterian Hospital at the end of 1943.

The pediatric service at CUMC (renamed in 2016 the Columbia University Irving Medical Center) retained the Babies Hospital name for several decades until the hospital was renamed the Babies and Children's Hospital in 1994 and renamed again the Morgan Stanley Children's Hospital of New York-Presbyterian in 2003 (reflecting the donation of an investment bank which permitted the construction of a new building and home for the hospital). Renaming medical centers and their associated institutions in order to honor rich patrons has become a commonplace in academic medicine in the United States. Whatever the name, Babies Hospital has served as the core of the Department of Pediatrics of the Columbia University College of Physicians and Surgeons (renamed the Columbia University Vagelos College of Physicians and Surgeons in 2017) for almost a century.

And Martha Wollstein should have been promoted to professor.

Rustin McIntosh

Rustin McIntosh was destined to be a star in academic medicine: he certainly had the credentials.

He was born in Omaha, Nebraska, in 1894, and his family moved to Yonkers in 1903. Rustin's mother taught him how to play the piano, and he spent 6 months in Germany and Switzerland at the age of 13 in order to learn German and French. He graduated at 16 years of age from Phillips Exeter Academy in 1910 and Harvard College in 1914 with a B.A., magna cum laude. He completed Harvard Medical School in 1918 at 24 years of age, earning an M.D., again magna cum laude; he was elected both to Phi Beta Kappa and Alpha Omega Alpha. After service in the US Army Medical Corps in World War I (including the award of a Croix de Guerre), he returned to train as an intern in pathology at Boston City Hospital in 1920, then as an intern in Internal Medicine at the Presbyterian Hospital in New York City, and finally as an intern and resident in Pediatrics at Babies Hospital (at this time still located on Manhattan's East Side at Lexington and 55th St.) through 1923. His mentor at Babies Hospital was Luther Emmett Holt, Sr.

McIntosh was not yet 30 years old when Holt decided that McIntosh was the best person available to lead Babies Hospital after his own retirement. Holt recommended him in glowing terms: "He is a man whom we must attach strongly to the hospital ... by all odds he is the most promising man for future advancement." Holt died in 1924 while on a trip to China, leaving McIntosh without a mentor. In spite of his background, McIntosh was then unsure how best to continue his academic pursuits.

In a letter to Helen Taussig (at Johns Hopkins) in 1970, McIntosh described what happened next:

Early in 1927 I decided to give up practice in New York City and consulted with my friend Bill Palmer (Walter W. Palmer) who at that time was head of the department of Internal Medicine at Columbia. Most wisely he advised me *not* to go abroad, as the fashion had been up to then, but to seek a position under one of the three men he considered to be the outstanding pediatricians: Ned Park, Kenneth Blackfan, and McKim Marriott. Largely on the basis of a brief meeting with Ned when he visited Babies Hospital during my residency (about 1923), I put him first among the three, and went up to New Haven to ask for a job. Though I was greatly helped by his intimate friendship with Bill Palmer, he told me with regret that he didn't have a vacant position (he knew then that he'd be moving to Hopkins in the autumn, and the size of his staff was largely controlled by the University's budget for pediatrics), but that there was a rumor current that Ethel Luce, of his Yale staff, was thinking of getting married; and if she did, I might have her place. To my immense good fortune Lucy did indeed marry Sam Clausen in time for me to close out my practice and join Ned's staff in Baltimore in October 1927. By such tenuous threads are our destinies suspended. [7]

Ned Park was Edwards A. Park: he had also been an intern under Holt and took over as Pediatrician-in-Chief of the Harriet Lane Home[10] of Johns Hopkins in 1927. Park wrote of McIntosh nearly three decades later: "One did not have to be with him long before realizing the rapidity of his uptake, his splendid qualities as observer and diagnostician, and his excellent judgement" [7].

McIntosh remained at Hopkins from late 1927 until early 1930, and though the threads appeared perhaps a bit tenuous to himself (he was not prone to self-aggrandizement, but had no lack of self-confidence), Holt's recommendation was eventually heeded. To no one else's surprise, McIntosh accepted a professorship in Pediatrics at Columbia University, though he almost immediately decided to visit many of the major European children's hospitals (in spite of his friend Palmer's counsel):

Before taking over the reins [at Babies Hospital], he was granted a year's leave of absence. It was a profitable year, beginning with several months in England, mostly at Cambridge, followed by a tour of the pediatric centers of the continent. He established relationships with many of the leading figures in European pediatrics, many of which were sustained in later years. [7]

Officially he was Professor of Diseases in Children (on leave) at Columbia University until July 1, 1931. He then assumed the title of Carpentier Professor of

---

[10] A medical clinic dedicated to children.

Fig. 6.4 Rustin McIntosh
late in his career at Babies
Hospital. (Courtesy of the
National Library of
Medicine)

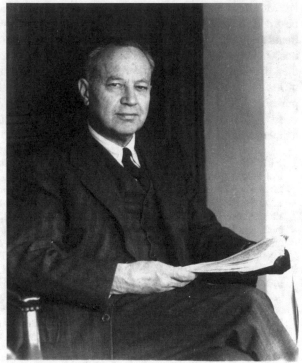

Diseases of Children at Columbia University and officially took over direction of
Babies Hospital. He was 37 years of age. Almost from his first day at Babies
Hospital, McIntosh helped provide an academic structure and direction for future
growth, and the Babies Hospital faculty – or at least most of them – were quickly
won over (Fig. 6.4).

It is worth considering how Wollstein must have felt about McIntosh's new academic rank in 1931: though he had published several interesting studies, none of his
work then or later approached the significance of Wollstein's work at the Rockefeller
Institute or at Babies Hospital. And in spite of Holt's recommendation and Park's
appreciation of his leadership skills, McIntosh had yet to make an impact as a leader
in academic pediatrics. Wollstein was never promoted beyond associate professor at
Columbia University, and she must have wondered how McIntosh had been recognized as a professor at such a young age: it may have appeared to her another example of the kind of gender bias which frustrated her at the Rockefeller Institute.

The move of Babies Hospital to its new home at CUMC occurred in 1929, little
more than a year before McIntosh took over as its Director (Fig. 6.5).

The hospital's move was perhaps less anxiety-provoking than were the changes
to its physician staff:

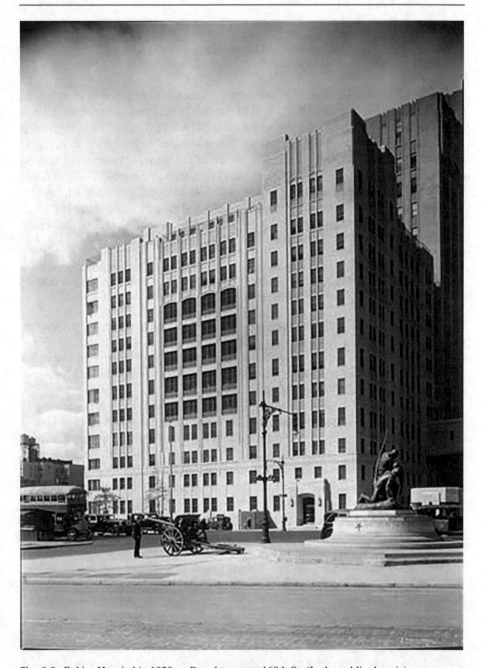

Fig. 6.5 Babies Hospital in 1929 on Broadway near 168th St. (In the public domain)

The group that arrived at the new location in June, 1929, was drawn from old Babies
Hospital, Bellevue and the erstwhile pediatric division of Presbyterian Hospital. From
Howard Mason (he was there and should know) we have the report that they all 'eyed each
other like strange cats in the same back yard' but gradually adjusted to each other. [21]

Babies Hospital was located on the same city block with Presbyterian Hospital, as
well as most of the rest of CUMC. Within a short time following the move, Babies
Hospital began to experience growing pains: it had over a hundred beds, a growing
physician staff, and a rapidly expanding interest in medical research. It began to
care for older children and adolescents. Some of the growing pains were also no
doubt associated with the onset of the Great Depression in October 1929, as noted
by Herbert Wilcox (the Medical Director of Babies Hospital preceding McIntosh):
"In spite of economic conditions, hospitals must and do continue to function" [21].

Moreover, the new connections to Presbyterian Hospital and Columbia University
actually proved valuable, as Rustin McIntosh noted:

What by some had been anticipated with manifest apprehension is now generally agreed to
have proved itself the means of emphasizing the capacity of the Babies Hospital both to
contribute to and profit from its association with other units of the Medical Center. [21]

It is likely that these connections helped stabilize the hospital's financial situation in
spite of dismal economic conditions generally. In addition, the gradual identification of Babies Hospital as an academic institution closely affiliated with Columbia
University had positive ramifications for the hospital's research and education activities, consistent with McIntosh's plans.

While McIntosh certainly encouraged excellence in his faculty, it is tempting to
suggest that he also had a genius for recognizing excellence, and this led him to
recruit a stellar group of pediatricians around him. The truth is, as usual, not so
simple. Several of the stars-to-be at Babies Hospital in the McIntosh Era were
already in place before McIntosh's tenure began (e.g., John Caffey, Ashley Weech,
and Martha Wollstein). And some of the stars-to-be were hired or recruited by
departments outside of McIntosh's purview (e.g., Virginia Apgar and Dorothy
Andersen). It is likely that McIntosh approved hiring Andersen as Assistant
Pathologist at Babies Hospital in 1935: he would certainly have been interested in
her, given her academic credentials as well as the recent conferral of a Columbia
University doctorate degree on her (though even in her new position at Babies
Hospital she was still employed by the University's Department of Pathology).
Nevertheless, McIntosh did recruit and hire several of the stars-to-be, including
Hattie Alexander and William Silverman, among many others.

Although McIntosh recognized and encouraged academic excellence in the
Babies Hospital faculty, the real source of his success was the mission he promoted:
pediatric care was at the apex of a pyramid supported by basic science and clinical
research, with a large helping of critical insight. The shared mission for the faculty
was to identify, as rapidly as possible, how to provide the best possible pediatric
care using contemporary scientific methods and then spread this new gospel to others. McIntosh was the leader who made it possible, and the Babies Hospital faculty
were loyal and responsive to his leadership. Douglas Damrosch noted about

McIntosh that: "Criticism when due is given quietly, even gently, but no less effectively for being gently given. He has always believed in a word to the wise; at most two or three words to the less wise" [22].

William Silverman credited McIntosh for his ability to motivate and engage the Babies Hospital faculty with his critical approach to medical care and research:

> I noticed that he was always able to see a whole elephant when those of us with lesser vision were arguing from the point of view of the animal's trunk, legs, or tail. He understood, full well that research questions are like blinders on a horse; they resist distraction, but they limit vision by removing the context in which meaning is embedded. The horse must remember to turn its head from time to time. [8]

Under McIntosh's direction, one of the defining characteristics at Babies Hospital was the development of a broad acceptance of this critical approach to medical care and research by the faculty. Silverman suggested that many of the faculty were "not team players" [23] and that as a result, opinions were judged on their merits, not on a speaker's perceived authority. Of course, judging an opinion on its merits at Babies Hospital during the McIntosh Era might demand more than the common ration of intellect and insight.

Early in his tenure, McIntosh developed a plan for Columbia University's Department of Pediatrics. As Damrosch noted:

> there is not much doubt that he (Dr. McIntosh) had a great deal to do with the improvement of morale. Indeed, his report [in 1933] did, I am convinced, mark the beginning of the esprit de corps for which Babies Hospital became widely known. [7]

This 1933 plan included both an assessment of the current status of the Department of Pediatrics at Columbia University with the attendant role of Babies Hospital and a blueprint for the future:

> It is clear that the Babies' Hospital as a physical plant will house the principal activities of the Department of Pediatrics... The medical staff of the hospital, outside of the resident intern staff, at present consists almost entirely of part-time men well equipped to care for patients but on the whole poorly equipped for investigative work. To foster the latter, I hope to bring to the Department men who are attracted to full-time intramural work by their interest in research.

McIntosh's frequent use of the male gender to describe a hospital staff which included women (in a hospital that was established by women) seems strange, but reflects the social norms of that era.

It may not always have been clear that Babies Hospital would play such a central role in Columbia University as suggested by McIntosh: after all, the hospital provided care only for infants and young children (while care for newborns was provided at CUMC's Sloane Hospital for Women, and care for adolescents was often provided at Presbyterian Hospital and at other CUMC affiliates). However, once this plan was committed to paper, it began to acquire an impetus and was eventually self-fulfilling: Babies Hospital gradually increased the age range of its patient population to include adolescents, and within a few years it encompassed all "the principal activities of the Department of Pediatrics" of Columbia University. Of course, this meant there was also an increased need for hospital space: for patients, for the medical staff responsible for patient care and teaching, and for research.

The first priority for space at Babies Hospital always went to patient care, while expanding research activities were limited principally by laboratory space: there was never enough room to permit routine, investigational, and basic science laboratory work to all be done on the scale envisioned by McIntosh within the hospital. McIntosh pointed out in 1939:

> At the time the present building of Babies Hospital was designed, it was the understanding that all the pediatric laboratories, both those designed for research and those intended for routine determinations, were to be housed within these walls. [24]

However there was never enough building space to accommodate this "understanding."

The laboratories responsible for supporting patient care, for "routine determinations," were of primary importance:

> The diagnostic laboratories were all within Babies Hospital and each one of them was in close proximity to its supervising pediatrician. Also, and this was of singular importance, each was immediately available to senior staff, house staff, and students who could easily drop by. [25]

Physician education was thus included as a part of the mission of the laboratories responsible for supporting patient care,[11] and research of any kind – clinical or basic science – was relegated to third place behind patient care and physician education. Babies Hospital laboratories were ultimately required to perform several functions simultaneously and to do all this in a very limited space.

McIntosh also knew there was no available space for the department of pediatrics in the adjacent medical school campus [24], and it was obvious that a conflict regarding insufficient research space at Babies Hospital would sooner or later emerge into the open (as it did in 1949). One of McIntosh's possible solutions – which he recommended subject to Wollstein's approval in 1933 – is particularly interesting to consider in the context of Dorothy Andersen's career: "Transference of the department of pathology of the Babies' Hospital to the Medical School, with liberation of the present pathological laboratory space for research purposes" [7]. McIntosh later thought better of this (or perhaps Wollstein convinced him it was not a good idea, or perhaps he rapidly became convinced of Andersen's value to the

---

[11] In 1935, Hattie Alexander supervised the bacteriology lab, Ashley Weech the chemistry lab, and Beryl Paige the pathology lab. In the last few decades of the twentieth century, hospital diagnostic labs have been tightly regulated to improve quality and accuracy, and clinicians no longer routinely supervise hospital labs: the only labs available to clinicians in most academic medical centers are research labs, usually dependent upon external funding. These labs are often located apart from the hospital (due in large part to the persistent problem of insufficient space). The participation of clinicians in lab testing and supervision is now mainly of historical interest only (though the progressive growth of bedside lab testing may eventually help obviate the loss).

Department of Pediatrics), and pediatric pathology remained at Babies Hospital throughout his tenure.

To implement the rest of his 1933 plan, McIntosh needed political skills which would allow him to obtain additional resources from the medical school, the medical center, and outside the university; of course, he needed to do all this without squandering any of the available resources already belonging to Babies Hospital. His interpersonal skills served him well; he was perceived as someone who was:

> capable of negotiating interdepartmental associations without compromising independence. During subsequent years, Rusty demonstrated his genius for soothing friction, mediating wrangles, avoiding predations and, when necessary as a last resort, engaging would-be predators in open combat. [25]

In 1932 shortly after joining Babies Hospital, McIntosh married Millicent Carey, the head of the Brearley School in New York City. She later was named Dean and later the first President of Barnard College. They clearly qualified as a "power couple" in Manhattan: they were both intelligent, courageous, and gracious, and their chief concern seemed to be about living life to the fullest within the constraints of their professional careers. In the mid-1930s, they purchased a country home in Tyringham, Massachusetts (in the Berkshires), and spent summers there with their family (including eventually five children), playing classical chamber music, gardening, and hiking.

By the late 1930s, much of the character of Babies Hospital during the McIntosh Era was firmly established. Inpatient care responsibilities were described by Douglas Damrosch:

> Three ward floors housed pediatric patients, one for infants, one for toddlers and one for older children—all being cared for by the pediatric house staff with the guidance of the attending pediatricians. But there were other floors that were assigned to other services: surgery, urology and otolaryngology. These were primarily the responsibility of the appropriate staffs but to each was assigned a pediatric resident, a collaboration which enhanced patient care as well as house staff training. For the most part this worked well but there were occasional interdepartmental disagreements, sometimes heated ones that ultimately required Rusty's intervention in the form of a conference between the two directors. Rusty's quiet manner calmed things down and the problem more often than not was resolved expeditiously. [25]

Sounds easy, but of course it wasn't: excellent clinical care required the collaboration of many, coupled with inspired leadership. Limited laboratory space persisted as a chronic problem. And academic success as envisioned by McIntosh was actually dependent, in the final analysis, on exceptional individuals. Andersen was one of those individuals who were vital to the academic success of Babies Hospital, and her career spanned all three decades of the McIntosh Era.

But there were others, and several of them were women.

References

1. Horn SS, Goetz CG. The election of Sarah McNutt as the first woman member of the American Neurological Association. Neurology. 2002;59(1):113–7.
2. Markel H. Academic pediatrics: the view of New York City a century ago. Acad Med. 1996;71(2):146–51.
3. McNutt SJ. Medical women, yesterday and today. Med Rec. 1918;94(4):135–9.
4. Dunn PM. Dr Emmett Holt (1855–1924) and the foundation of North American paediatrics. Arch Dis Child Fetal Neonatal Ed. 2000;83(3):F221–3.
5. Mason HH, Park EA. Luther Emmet Holt, 1855-1924. J Pediatr. 1956;49(3):342–69.
6. Dawson P. Dorothy in a man's world. North Charleston: CreateSpace Independent Publishing Platform; 2016.
7. Rustin McIntosh papers. Archives at the Augustus C. Long Health Sciences Library of Columbia University.
8. Silverman WA. In search of the spirit of Babies Hospital. In: Babies Hospital, editor. Babies Hospital historical collection, 1887–1994. Archives at the Augustus C. Long Health Sciences Library of Columbia University.
9. Babies Hospital historical archives. Archives at the Augustus C. Long Health Sciences Library of Columbia University.
10. Straus J, Strauss L. Rusty McIntosh by some of the many who experienced the essence of his presence at Babies Hospital, 1931–1960. Babies Hospital Alumni Association; 1987.
11. Bryan CS, Podolsky SH. Sir William Osler (1849-1919) – the uses of history and the singular beneficence of medicine. N Engl J Med. 2019;381(23):2194–6.
12. Wright JR Jr, Abrams J. Martha Wollstein of Babies Hospital in New York City (1868-1939)-the first North American pediatric pathologist. Pediatr Dev Pathol. 2018;21(5):437–43.
13. Sicherman B, Green CH. Notable American women: the modern period: a biographical dictionary. Cambridge, MA: The Belknap Press of Harvard University Press; 1980.
14. Lancefield R. AAI looks back: PI in the Scotland Yard of streptococcal mysteries. 2013. Available from: https://www.aai.org/AAISite/media/About/History/Articles/AAI_History_009.pdf.
15. Abrams J, Wright JR Jr. Martha Wollstein: a pioneer American female clinician-scientist. J Med Biogr. 2020;28(3):168–74.
16. Wollstein M. PFEIFFER'S BACILLUS AND INFLUENZA: A SEROLOGICAL STUDY. J Exp Med. 1919;30(6):555–68.
17. Wollstein M, Spence RC. A study of tuberculosis in infants and young children. Am J Dis Child. 1921;21(1):48–56.
18. Wollstein M, Bartlett FH. A study of tuberculous lesions in infants and young children, based on post-mortem examinations. Am J Dis Child. 1914;VIII(5):362–76.
19. Wollstein M, Bartlett FH. Brain tumors in young children: a clinical and pathologic study. Am J Dis Child. 1923;25(4):257–83.
20. M. R. Martha Wollstein, M.D. 1868-1939. Am J Dis Child. 1939;58(6):1301–1.
21. McIntosh R. The McIntosh era at Babies Hospital, 1931–1960: a commemorative volume to honor Rustin McIntosh. Babies Hospital; 1960.
22. Damrosch DS. Highlight-Rustin McIntosh. Alumni Association Bulletin, College of Physicians and Surgeons, Columbia University; 1961. VI.
23. Silverman WA. Oral history project: William A. Sliverman, MD, L.M. Gartner, Editor. American Academy of Pediatrics; 1997.
24. Annual report of the Babies Hospital of the City of New York. New York: The Babies Hospital of the City of New York; 1889–1942.
25. Damrosch DS. A tribute to Rustin McIntosh, M.D., C.-P.M. Center, Editor. 1986.

Synergy

On July 1, 1935, Martha Wollstein retired as Pathologist of Babies Hospital after almost 45 years of service. Her replacement was Beryl Paige, and Andersen then took Paige's position as Assistant Pathologist. Andersen was 34 years old, and she was first identified as the responsible pathologist for a pediatric autopsy at Babies Hospital in August.

In September 1935 Andersen performed an autopsy on a 10-year-old girl who was admitted with epiglottitis; she remained hospitalized until her death four months later from pneumonia and meningitis[1] due to *Haemophilus influenzae*.[2] She was the first patient in the United States to be treated with an antibiotic [1]. At autopsy, Andersen noted both acute and subacute *Haemophilus influenzae* meningitis. The acute component consisted of the recent development of a new exudate (i.e., pus) in the subarachnoid space surrounding the brain, while the subacute component was consistent with the original infection a month or more earlier.

Up until this time, the mortality rate for *Haemophilus influenzae* meningitis was nearly 100%. Martha Wollstein, who first recognized the importance of this bacteria in pediatric meningitis, had suggested several decades earlier that antiserum (containing antibodies against *Haemophilus influenzae* collected from goats) was helpful in treating a simian model of this disease [2], but progress in adapting this therapy to humans was slow after she left the Rockefeller Institute: follow-up reports suggested that this immunologic therapy (antiserum from an animal source) might be only partially effective.

Ashley Weech was the attending physician responsible for this patient. Weech was an epicurean, fond of wine, fishing, and "appreciation for the good things in life" [3], but he was also a highly accomplished academic physician who later chaired the Department of Pediatrics at the University of Cincinnati:

---

[1] Meningitis is an infection of the fluid and membranes surrounding the brain and spinal cord.

[2] A type of bacteria which may cause epiglottitis, meningitis, pneumonia, and sepsis.

His fame as a teacher of pediatrics reached international proportions as did the department that he headed. His research interests includes fundamental knowledge on the permeability of membranes, plasma proteins, edema, and nutrition. He served as president of the American Pediatric Society and he was given the Borden and Jacobi Awards as well as a Distinguished Service Medal from the Columbia-Presbyterian Medical Center.

Following the request of the patient's physician father, who had searched the medical literature looking for anything which might help his deathly ill daughter, Weech had arranged with a pharmaceutical firm to obtain a small quantity of sulfachrysoidine (a sulfonamide antibiotic) for a 13-day course of treatment. Though unsuccessful at saving her life, antibiotic therapy seemed to have been associated with some transient improvement, both in her fever and in her overall clinical condition (after a few days of antibiotic therapy, her neurosurgeon noted that "this child looks better today than at any time since I have seen her [1]"). In addition, cultures of the cerebrospinal fluid obtained during her illness were negative until nearly two months following antibiotic treatment (and only a few days prior to her death), when *Haemophilus influenzae* was isolated: it was possible that the antibiotic had been partially effective, helping to explain Andersen's findings at autopsy.

Hattie Alexander had been on the faculty of Babies Hospital for a few years by then, and Andersen's autopsy results would have been of great interest to her. Alexander graduated from Johns Hopkins Medical School in 1930 (four years after Andersen) and then completed an internship at the Harriet Lane Home from 1930 to 1931, and in 1931, Rustin McIntosh (whom Alexander knew at Hopkins) invited her to pursue further training at Babies Hospital: she agreed, landing there at the beginning of the McIntosh Era. She was awarded the Holt Fellowship in Diseases of Children (once held by McIntosh) in 1932, and following that she joined the faculty of Babies Hospital during the last few years of Wollstein's career. It is likely that McIntosh was thinking of Alexander when he remarked about Wollstein that "with those who sought her [Wollstein's] help … she eagerly shared her wide store of knowledge with open generosity" [4]: Alexander began to investigate bacterial meningitis early in her career at Babies Hospital, and Wollstein would likely have offered her mentorship. Andersen's autopsy results must also have been a stimulus to Alexander: her research agenda then began to focus more specifically on bacterial meningitis.

In 1937 (2 years after the death of the 10-year-old girl with *Haemophilus influenzae* meningitis), Alexander's first two publications appeared: both were investigations on the utility of equine antiserum to help diagnose meningococcal meningitis [5, 6]. Her coauthor on one of these studies [6] and contributor to the other [5] was Geoffrey Rake of the Rockefeller Institute: he had joined the Institute several years after Wollstein left, and his work helped establish the role of different strains of meningococcus in epidemics of meningitis. Though Alexander was never officially affiliated with the Rockefeller Institute, her work over several years suggested shared goals with several of the Institute's researchers.[3]

---

[3] Alexander's work on antiserum and bacterial disease was in large part a continuation of work by Wollstein, Rake, and Oswald Avery at the Institute and culminated in her collaboration with former

Following Wollstein's earlier insights, Alexander reported in 1939 that rabbit (not goat or horse) antiserum to *Haemophilus influenzae* "yielded encouraging results in the treatment of children with H. influenzal meningitis" [7]. She eventually showed greatly improved survival of children with *Haemophilus influenzae* meningitis who were treated with a sulfonamide antibiotic and rabbit antiserum (when indicated) in 1941 [8]: attacking this infection with both an antiserum and an antibiotic – each of which might be only partially effective – must have seemed like a much better idea than trying to use one or the other. This was a major therapeutic advance (and she received the E. Mead Johnson Award for it in 1943).

Alexander also noted about meningococcus in 1941 that "experimentally drug-resistant strains [to sulfanilamide[4]] are encountered frequently" [8]. Wollstein had described meningococcus resistance to antiserum decades earlier in 1914 using the effect of antiserum dilutions on agglutination [9], but the concept of antibiotic resistance was only beginning to emerge in the early 1940s, and Alexander played an important role in that new paradigm.

In 1946 Paul di Sant'Agnese and Dorothy Andersen were the first to report on the utility of penicillin therapy for CF patients with severe lung infections associated with *Staphylococcus aureus* (see Chap. 9), though they noted that some patients did not respond to penicillin due to apparent antibiotic resistance [10]. Their study included one patient (in late 1944) whose preterminal throat culture of *Staphylococcus aureus* showed resistance to penicillin which was further investigated at autopsy: "the organism was found to be resistant to a concentration of 250 units of penicillin per cubic centimeter" [10]. Alexander, who was by then the Director of the Bacteriology laboratory at Babies Hospital, was responsible for this result, including its expression as a dilution or concentration of the antibiotic.

A few months later, Alexander and her coinvestigator Grace Leidy were among the first to define antibiotic resistance using the concept of minimal effective concentration of an antibiotic in patients with *Haemophilus influenzae* meningitis treated with streptomycin [11, 12]. By 1947, Alexander and Leidy described the emergence of resistance as the result of a selective process, in which sensitive bacteria are killed off and resistant bacteria remain [13].

In sum, over several decades, the accomplishments of this influential trio of Babies Hospital physicians – Wollstein, Alexander, and Andersen – appear to have been synergistic (i.e., their combined efforts were greater than the sum of their separate efforts): consideration of the utility of antiserum in the treatment of bacterial meningitis, as well as resistance to antiserum by specific bacteria, and later of the utility of antibiotic treatment of bacterial meningitis and resistance to it by specific

---

Institute researcher Michael Heidelberger using antiserum to H*aemophilus influenzae* to treat meningitis associated with that bacterium. Her later work on the role of DNA in the transfer of genetic information in *Haemophilus influenzae* was a follow-up to the work of Avery's group at the Institute on the role of DNA in the transfer of genetic information in pneumococcus, while her later work on the role of RNA in the transfer of poliovirus genetic information seemed a continuation of work by Igor Tamm's group at the Institute. Alexander's career appeared to affirm the benefits of a (mostly informal) relationship with several of the Rockefeller Institute researchers.

[4]Another sulfonamide antibiotic.

bacteria were pursued over several decades by these researchers. How much did Alexander owe Wollstein for her early studies on immune therapy in bacterial meningitis and for the concept of resistance? What was the impact of Andersen's autopsy findings in 1935 on Alexander's subsequent research agenda? How much did Alexander contribute to Andersen's early recognition of penicillin resistance? It is likely that answers to these questions were unimportant to this trio of researchers: each contributed in some way to the other's accomplishments. Synergy in this situation reflects the collaborative and stimulating academic environment at Babies Hospital during the McIntosh Era. Importantly, Alexander's research efforts on the treatment of bacterial meningitis and antibiotic resistance were groundbreaking and helped launch her academic career.

In any case, Andersen had begun to establish a reputation of meticulous care and thoughtful analysis, and her expertise in pediatric pathology was quickly recognized. While her professional life was beginning to take shape, she began to work a bit on her private life as well.

References

1. Carithers HA. The first use of an antibiotic in America. Am J Dis Child. 1974;128(2):207–11.
2. Wollstein M. Serum treatment of influenzal meningitis. J Exp Med. 1911;14(1):73–82.
3. Ayoub EM. Introduction of Dr. A. Ashley Weech for the John Howland Award. From the American Pediatric Society, April 27, 1977, San Francisco, California. Pediatr Res. 1978;12(3):229–31.
4. M. R. Martha Wollstein, M.D. 1868–1939. Am J Dis Child. 1939;58(6):1301–1.
5. Alexander HE. Prognostic value of the precipitin test in meningococcus meningitis. J Clin Invest. 1937;16(2):207–11.
6. Alexander HE, Rake G. Studies on meningococcus infection: X. A further note on the presence of meningococcus precipitinogens in the cerebrospinal fluid. J Exp Med. 1937;65(3):317–21.
7. Alexander HE. Type "B" anti-influenzal rabbit serum for therapeutic purposes. Proc Soc Exp Biol Med. 1939;40(2):313–4.
8. Alexander HE. Treatment of bacterial meningitis. Bull N Y Acad Med. 1941;17(2):100–15.
9. Wollstein M. Parameningococcus and its antiserum. J Exp Med. 1914;20(3):201–17.
10. Di Sant'Agnese PA, Andersen DH. Celiac syndrome; chemotherapy in infections of the respiratory tract associated with cystic fibrosis of the pancreas; observations with penicillin and drugs of the sulfonamide group, with special reference to penicillin aerosol. Am J Dis Child. 1946;72:17–61.
11. Alexander HE, Leidy G, et al. Hemophilus influenzae meningitis treated with streptomycin. J Am Med Assoc. 1946;132:434–40.
12. Gilsdorf JR. Continual raving: a history of meningitis and the people who conquered it. Oxford University Press; 2019.
13. Alexander HE, Leidy G. Mode of action of streptomycin on type b H. influenzae: 1. Origin of resistant organisms. J Exp Med. 1947;85(4):329–38.

Andy's Abandoned Farm

8

Dorothy Andersen's dedication to work meant that she was more than willing to spend long hours each day testing hypotheses in a pathology laboratory or reviewing medical literature in a library: as a student, she had developed an overriding interest in "laboratory experimentation," and she continued to apply that approach to her work as a pathologist. However devotion to hard work is difficult to maintain for long stretches of time; without friends and time off for relaxation, devotion to work is liable to be a lonely and frustrating endeavor.

While Andersen was mostly successful at keeping her private life private,[1] she had numerous friends throughout her career: some were her colleagues at work, while many others had no connection with healthcare or academic medicine. Almost all of them – along with their families – were Andersen's guests at one time or another on a remote hillside in northwestern New Jersey.

In 1938 [1, 2] Andersen became the proud owner of some land adjacent to High Point State Park near the Delaware River: she purchased 100 acres for eight dollars an acre from Robert Norris [1]. The land and its buildings were described decades after Andersen's death as "Andy's abandoned farm" [2]. Back in 1938, the only buildings on the site were in great need of repair and included "a barn, a lean-to, and an outhouse" [1, 2]. At least for the first few years, amenities were few: no running water or electricity and heat provided by a single wood-burning stove. Andersen noted that it was "a small rocky farm on a hill, where I have rebuilt a couple of humble buildings into a week-end camp- a strenuous job for self and friends, all of us starting in ignorance of carpentry" [3]. Though its beginnings were humble, the

---

[1] In response to a question in 1944 from Mt. Holyoke's alumni office "Name and address of person most likely always to know your whereabouts," Andersen responded with: "?". In 1947 she answered the same question with: "Babies Hospital." Though this might suggest a lonely private life with little, if any, time off for relaxation, it is more likely a reflection of her complicated and busy life: many of her close friends were aware of some of her activities, but she didn't share all the details of both her public and private lives with anyone.

© The Author(s), under exclusive license to Springer Nature Switzerland AG 2022
J. S. Baird, *Dorothy Hansine Andersen*,
https://doi.org/10.1007/978-3-030-87484-1_8

resulting "week-end camp"[2] developed into more than just an abandoned farm, and it became the center of Andersen's life away from work. The barn was converted into a house, and the house eventually included a chimney with two fireplaces and a kitchen.

The skills required of Andersen in this effort were described years later:

> She was the head carpenter, the chief mason, the one who knew how to trim oil lamps, sharpen a chain saw, cut grass with a scythe, or charm an old one-lunger engine into running in order to cut wood with a belt-driven table saw. [1]

Andersen "found relaxation in hard manual labor and satisfaction in the skilled use of her hands" [4], as she built a fireplace and a kitchen chimney, lay floors, and cut lots of firewood. She was assisted by students, physicians-in-training, and friends, but she cheerfully bore the brunt of this labor, all the while also cooking meals for her numerous guests.

In order to be comfortable during a visit to the abandoned farm, Andersen and her friends needed enough wood to burn in the stove and fireplaces almost constantly, as well as an abundant supply of fresh water from a spring about a quarter of a mile distant. These were the bare essentials critical to maintain at any time of the year:

> Even in mid-summer, the large barn-like structure seemed impervious to sun. A Franklin stove in the kitchen ran constantly, replacing dampness with warmth, and radiating heat immediately upward. Those not lucky enough to be assigned the toasty upstairs bedroom, at nighttime pulled a heated brick from the oven, wrapped it in a towel, and carried it to bed with them. [5]

Whatever hardships guests had to undergo were actually part of the farm's appeal: the hardships were shared, and they contributed to the stories her guests and friends told each other about their visits. Celia Ores remembered that farm guests were given tasks: Ores' task usually involved picking vegetables and fruit from the garden to include in meals and drinks [6, 7], while others were tasked with fetching water and cutting wood (Fig. 8.1).

Andersen described the abandoned farm as "a primitive retreat well hidden in the Kittittinny Range of northwest New Jersey.... It is also a fine place for birds, photography, sketching, cooking, eating, and conversation" [3]. This farm may have reminded her a bit of the farm in Vermont where her father's family lived or of the Massey farm; perhaps it even recalled stories from her father's family about Bornholm in Denmark. Andersen's Holyoke classmate Marion Beman Chute's poem "Abandoned Farm" described some of its charms:

> If you should walk the overgrown old roads
>   All 'round the mountain, every now and then

---

[2] Margaret (Peg) Miller, daughter of Marion Beman Chute, noted that her family first visited the farm in May 1948 when Miller was 6 years old; her family "continued going on weekends once a month and for 2 or 3 week summer vacations until 1955."

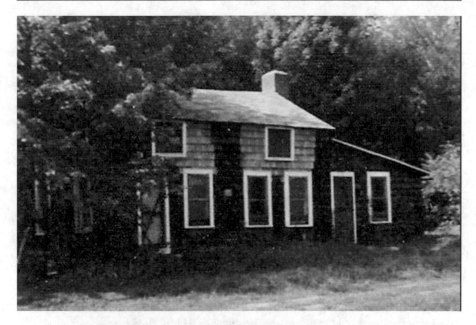

Fig. 8.1 Andersen's converted barn at her farm. (In the public domain)

> You'd come upon a lilac, snowball bush
> Or Yellow rose that says folks lived there once,
> And find the cellar holes, perhaps a dozen,
> Each with a story that we'll never know. [8]

Chute noted the large variety of wildlife which frequented the farm, including bears, chipmunks, deer, fisher cats, porcupines, rabbits, raccoons, salamanders, skunks, snakes, woodchucks, and numerous birds and fishes; she also described the sometimes humorous interactions between farm guests and wildlife. She concluded:

> Yes, wildness up to now's been coming back
>   For forty years.[3] But can it last much longer
> This near the city? What a loss 'twould be
> If seasons passed and there were no arbutus,
> No lady's slipper and no cardinal flower;
> If June came on without its evening chorus
> (Wood thrushes 'twas when we first came, but now
> Veeries sing spirals. Once I heard a hermit);
> Or toward mid-August, when the birds fall silent,
> No katydids tuned up to take their place;
> And we should never hear from out the darkness
> The owl's deep-voiced "Hoohoo, hoohoo, hoohoo"! [8]

Chute's celebration of nature at the abandoned farm also emphasized the culinary joys of the farm's fish and fruit trees and of the berries and produce from the kitchen

---

[3] This suggests that the poem was written in the late 1970s.

garden, and it recalls somewhat Thomas Wolfe's celebration of Asheville during Andersen's childhood.

Andy's abandoned farm served as a refuge not just for wildlife and for Andersen and her friends but also for the next generation of her friends' families. Andersen and her friends passed their vacations and holidays there, shared the simple pleasures of a rural existence away from work, and were witness to the changing seasons. Even in winter, the abandoned farm had guests: "the year 1939 dragged to a close, with Hilde[4] spending what had now become a tradition of eggnog, New Year's day, warm friendships- all the ingredients of a perfect winter break- at Andersen's farm" [5]. Andersen and her guests played games [1, 5],[5] learned about carpentry and masonry, and hiked in the surrounding countryside. Her farm represented in part the Vermont tradition that was an important part of her personality; it was also a reminder and an affirmation of her deep appreciation for the natural world.

Around the same time that Andersen purchased the farm, she also became a member of the Appalachian Mountain Club; this was one of the first groups to mix outdoor recreation with environmental activism, similar to the Sierra Club. Andersen's appreciation of conservation and her interest in and respect for the natural world dated back at least to her undergraduate years, if not earlier. The farm and the Appalachian Mountain Club helped her to reclaim some of her earliest passions, extending back even to the summers she spent as a child in Vermont.

A visit to Andy's abandoned farm in the spring of 2021[6] was only possible via a little-used, unmarked dirt road, followed by a short walk – no more than a hundred yards or so – to a remote clearing in the woods just west of High Point State Park: the buildings are all gone, their positions marked by two chimneys no more than fifty yards apart. The older chimney is the one Andersen and her friends built for the barn which they converted into a house by 1940; this chimney was made both of bricks and stones, but only the stone base remains. The converted barn burned down over a decade after Andersen's death [1], and a second chimney was then built for a converted "shack" – another primitive structure converted into a second residence on the abandoned farm. This "shack" eventually became a "snugly paneled guest house" with accommodations for eight, though it too eventually fell into disrepair and had to be dismantled and removed [8]. The second chimney is almost all stone and seems to be a bit sturdier than the first chimney. Near the second chimney is a cellar hole, and a narrow creek runs a few yards east into a small dam no more than a few feet high, constructed of crumbling stones and cement. This creek – named Brook Minor by Andersen – feeds into a pool no bigger than a bathtub just a few yards in front of the dam, though the pool is gradually filling in with branches and stones.[7]

---

[4] Hilde Bruch, a pediatrician and a refugee from Nazi Germany, later a psychiatrist at CUMC, was a close friend and a frequent guest at the farm (often accompanied by her mother and her nephew Herbert). She later became one of the foremost experts on eating disorders.

[5] In Hilde Bruch's biography, Andersen "soon discovered that she had much in common with her colleague's [Hilde Bruch's] nephew [Herbert]. Both loved games- any games: cards, chess, match it, pick up sticks- whatever they knew or could invent, they did with fervor."

[6] Arranged and with the generous guidance of Martin Rapp of the New Jersey Natural Lands Trust.

[7] Biographer's note: however it still tempted my dog to a quick swim. When I dried her off later I discovered she had picked up dozens of ticks.

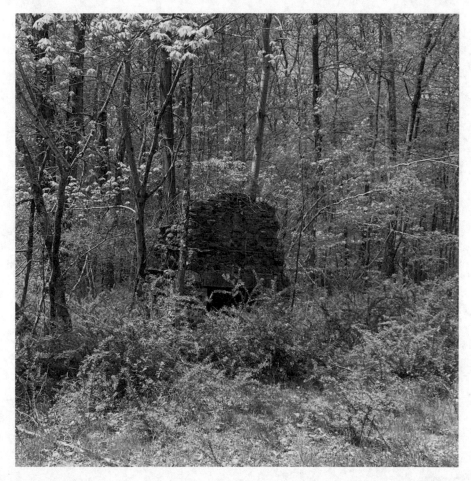

Fig. 8.2 The remains of Andersen's chimney which she built for the converted barn. (Photo by JS Baird, 2021)

Nature has indeed begun to reclaim the site, as suggested in Chute's poem, though the oaks and hickory characteristic of the original forests here will take decades to return. Chestnut saplings have reappeared [2] following the blight over a century ago, but they also will require time to mature. Evidence of wildlife around the abandoned farm persists: bear scat in the grassy clearing, a garter snake sunning itself on some gravel, and tree trunks gnawed by porcupines. There were, however, also a few flowers that seemed to recall Andersen: a patch of narcissus and a bushy rose between the creek and the clearing. While it was a pleasantly warm spring day closer to the coast, a light jacket was helpful at the abandoned farm. It was obvious that Andersen and her farm guests were a hardy bunch (Fig. 8.2).

In 1938, the same year she purchased the farm, Andersen published the results of several years of meticulous work on a select group of infants and children with celiac disease: her recognition and description of a new disease she called "cystic fibrosis of the pancreas" in these patients was a momentous occasion, which she celebrated at her farm.

References

1. Miller MP. History of Andy's farm, M. Rapp, Editor. 2013.
2. New Jersey Natural Lands Trust, editor. New Jersey Natural Lands Trust: 2013 annual report. Trenton: New Jersey Natural Lands Trust. 2013.
3. Dorothy H. Andersen papers. Archives at the Augustus C. Long Health Sciences Library of Columbia University.
4. Damrosch DS. Dorothy Hansine Andersen. J Pediatr. 1964;65:477–9.
5. Bruch JH. Unlocking the Golden cage: an intimate biography of Hilde Bruch, M.D. Gürze Books; 1996.
6. Ores C. Interview with Celia Ores, J.S. Baird, Editor. 2021.
7. Ores C. Reading Pushkin in Siberia. Lulu Publishing Services; 2016.
8. Chute MB. Abandoned farm (a poem). In: New Jersey Natural Lands Trust: 2013 annual report. 2013.

Scoring the First Goal

9

It cannot have escaped Dorothy Andersen's notice that Martha Wollstein, now recognized as one of the founders of pediatric pathology [1], faded quickly from view:

> Her colleagues seldom got to know her as a person. Many considered her difficult to work with; few bothered to pierce the protective shell of this intellectually gifted, shy, and lonely woman. Following her retirement in 1935, she moved to Grand Rapids, Michigan. She returned to New York in 1939 to enter the Mount Sinai Hospital as a patient and died there that September. She was buried in Beth-El Cemetery, Brooklyn. Her death, like her life, was hardly noticed. A handful of colleagues attended her funeral, and obituary notices were brief --at best a paltry witness to the achievement of this distinguished pioneer in pediatric pathology. [2]

Depressing. Anyone considering a similar career path might want to reconsider. Though Wollstein's influence and accomplishments persisted among those few who knew and worked with her, her mentorship contributed to accomplishments after she was gone, and her career seemed at first glance to be a model for other women, it was disconcerting how quickly her prestige disappeared.

Andersen began to develop some potential research interests during her first few years as a pathologist and began to search for a way to use those interests in order to make important contributions to medical science which might not fade. Chronic lung disease was common in her autopsy work on adults at Presbyterian Hospital: was this occasionally the result of some unknown childhood disease? As there were still not enough available medical tools to enable an adequate investigation of this hypothesis, it is likely she set this question aside for later. However, as chance does seem to favor the prepared mind, it is likely that some of her early work on adults with chronic lung disease helped prepare her for her later work on "cystic fibrosis of the pancreas." An example from one of her autopsies in 1929 at Presbyterian Hospital is particularly relevant:

- A 34-year-old "Irishman" died after a 10-day hospitalization for pneumonia. He had previous hospitalizations for pneumonia, hemoptysis, and lung abscess and

J. S. Baird, *Dorothy Hansine Andersen*,
https://doi.org/10.1007/978-3-030-87484-1_9

a history of a chronic cough with purulent sputum. On admission, his fingernails were clubbed, and he had acrocyanosis, as well as signs of right-sided pneumonia with a collection of pleural fluid. His sputum culture grew *Staphylococcus aureus*. Pus from the right pleural space was drained (via a thoracotomy). On autopsy there was extensive bronchiectasis with adenomas in the pancreas and nearly absent spermatozoa with an obstructed epididymis.

It is possible that this patient had a milder type of "cystic fibrosis of the pancreas" permitting survival to adulthood, though no one could have known this at the time. Andersen may have retained some awareness of this symptom complex, as chance favors the prepared mind.

She had also been intrigued by heart disease in adults, and she found abnormal hearts in infants and children equally fascinating, as was any kind of liver disease. Children with celiac disease at Babies Hospital also quickly caught her interest: we now believe it to be an autoimmune disease affecting mainly the small intestine, in which symptoms are associated with gluten ingestion and typically lead to malabsorption, though this was all unknown in the 1930s when celiac disease was diagnosed by the presence of symptoms. For much of the twentieth century, there was no specific therapy.

It would have been more accurate at that time to designate celiac disease as a syndrome: a syndrome is a collection of signs and symptoms associated with one or more diseases, while a disease requires a specific causal mechanism. Andersen came to believe that a careful investigation of patients with a particular syndrome might permit the identification of a new disease (or several new diseases) which would then be considered separately from the syndrome.

The index case for Andersen's landmark 1938 CF study was a child who died on November 24, 1935 (case 44 [3]), only two months after Andersen's autopsy of the ten year-old child with *Haemophilus influenzae* meningitis (not eighteen months later, as suggested elsewhere [4]). Andersen later wrote that "it happened that a child who had presented the clinical picture of celiac disease came to post-mortem examination and was found to have a lesion in the pancreas now known as cystic fibrosis" [5]. This unfortunate three year old girl was admitted in early November for an operation to treat congenital torticollis: cutting (dividing) the right sternocleidomastoid muscle to prevent her head from constantly turning to the left. She was malnourished (weight below the fifth percentile for age), and her diet had been modified for celiac disease (she received a low-starch/low-fat diet with supplemental milk and bananas). Following surgery, she developed pneumonia and died three weeks later.[1]

At autopsy, purulent bronchitis, pneumonia, and lung abscesses (particularly in the right middle lobe) associated with *Staphylococcus aureus* were present, along

---

[1] Any suggestion that Andersen had seen this patient in 1934 or earlier (i.e., a year or more prior to Andersen's appointment at Babies Hospital) seems unlikely Andersen was then a pathologist affiliated with Presbyterian Hospital and did not then have any clinical responsibilities, in particular, for pediatric patients.

with hypertrophy of the right side of the heart. Andersen noted that "a prolonged search for the pancreatic duct revealed only a small duct which extended 8 mm from the ampulla and was then lost in fibrous tissue" [3]. Microscopic examination of the pancreas revealed "dense fibrous tissue… [and] irregular clumps of tubules or cysts [3]" with preserved islets of Langerhans.[2] The scarred pancreatic tissue suggested a disturbance of pancreatic exocrine function: this meant that alkaline secretions from the pancreas containing the enzymes required for digestion of food were absent in this patient, but that pancreatic endocrine function was likely preserved.

Andersen's meticulous work as a pathologist was about to be surpassed by the gift of her clinical intuition, supported by her knowledge of physiology. For this first case of what she later identified as a new disease, Andersen insisted on a specific label in the hospital's autopsy records: "cystic fibrosis of the pancreas," and she speculated that the condition – as well as the absence of a pancreatic duct – might be congenital (Fig. 9.1).

This disease label was also used by Paige and others at Babies Hospital from December 1935 going forward in the hospital's autopsy records: the pancreas of any patient dying with celiac syndrome at Babies Hospital was then closely examined, and Andersen began to collect similar cases. She began to suspect that infants and children with an unknown disease characterized by this pancreatic lesion might include many of the infants and children who had celiac syndrome, in which malabsorption of various nutrients occurs; she now had a cause for malabsorption in a group of celiac syndrome patients, and she began to meticulously prepare the evidence for a study to allow recognition of this new disease.

An abnormal pancreas – with cysts and fibrosis present on microscopic examination alongside preserved islets of Langerhans – suggested pancreatic exocrine insufficiency, as noted above. She carefully reviewed the medical histories of all the infants and children she autopsied in order to ensure that pancreatic endocrine function was preserved, as she suspected. As she collected more cases, it was indeed clear that the pancreatic lesion in these patients involved exocrine function only and was present in at least some patients at birth or shortly afterward. It was also apparent that this lesion was associated with several distinct clinical presentations based on patient age at death. She suspected that useful comparisons might be made between patients with this new disease and those with celiac disease without pancreatic pathology.

She eventually collected forty-nine reports of pediatric autopsies with pancreatic cysts and fibrosis as well as clinical evidence of celiac syndrome (twenty from Babies Hospital, two from other hospitals, and twenty-seven from the medical literature), and reported this extended series in 1938 [3]. Much of the medical literature she reviewed was in German, including over a dozen of the cases she identified with this new disease. Andersen's expertise with foreign languages – not just German, but Italian and French as well – continued to be useful to her throughout her research career, as she relied on studies from many European medical journals

---

[2] These islets include the cells responsible for pancreatic endocrine function, including the secretion of hormones like insulin and glucagon.

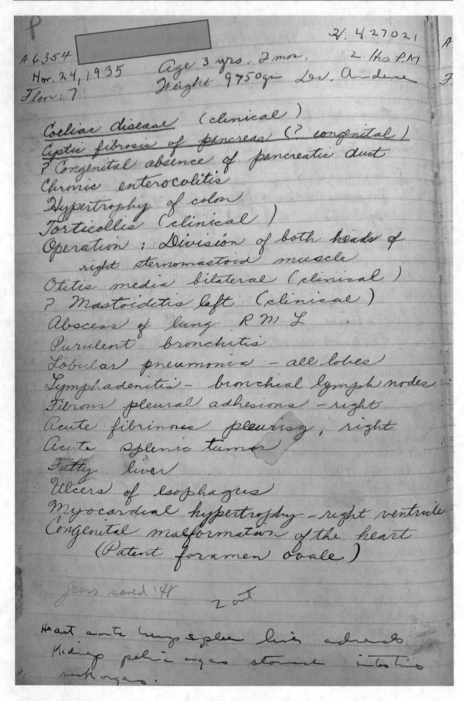

Fig. 9.1 The index patient with "cystic fibrosis of the pancreas" in the pathology register of autopsies at Babies Hospital in the 1930s. Andersen's spidery script is suggested by the scrawled "Dr. Andersen" in the upper right. (Photo by JS Baird, 2020)

to help support or illustrate her investigations. Following the traditions William Osler helped establish, Andersen presented meticulous, detailed case reports of the patients in her manuscript.

Andersen suggested that the infants and children with this new disease shared many of the symptoms of celiac syndrome; she suggested the descriptive name that she coined at Babies Hospital: "cystic fibrosis of the pancreas." She recognized that malabsorption with resultant growth failure – and occasional vitamin A[3] defi- ciency – was a particularly important problem associated with this new disease and suggested that insufficient pancreatic exocrine function was responsible. The obvi- ous implication of this suggestion was that a diagnostic strategy for the new disease might involve assessment of pancreatic exocrine function in patients whose symp- toms suggested celiac syndrome. Andersen also noted that the clinical type of mal- absorption affecting many infants and children with this new disease seemed to be fat malabsorption, potentially explaining vitamin A deficiency in these patients.

Andersen noted age-related changes in the disease pattern: neonates (five of the forty-nine cases) died with bowel obstruction, occasionally associated with meco- nium ileus and/or peritonitis.[4] Infants up to the age of six months (nineteen of the forty-nine cases) died with failure to thrive and lung infections; their course was often characterized by chronic cough. Older infants and children (twenty-five of the forty-nine cases; the oldest was fourteen years of age) were all malnourished and died with lung disease (purulent bronchitis, pneumonia, and/or bronchiectasis, often associated with *Staphylococcus aureus*), occasionally with a fatty liver and cirrho- sis. These age-related clinical manifestations of cystic fibrosis (CF) have been con- sistently validated over the decades since Andersen's study.

Seven of the twenty-seven cases that she abstracted from the medical literature with "cystic fibrosis of the pancreas" also had a diagnosis of vitamin A deficiency, including four cases from a report by Kenneth Blackfan and Burt Wolbach in 1933 [6]. Vitamin A is not well-absorbed in patients with fat malabsorption, and a defi- ciency is associated with epithelial cell[5] abnormalities similar to those found by Andersen in the airways of some of the patients with CF. She suggested that these changes in epithelial cells might conceivably be associated with an increased risk of infection. It therefore seemed possible to her that vitamin A deficiency might be responsible for lung infection and disease in these patients. Andersen continued to ponder this possibility for several years. In her 1938 study she suggested that "pul- monary infection was possibly secondary to vitamin A deficiency."

---

[3] One of the fat-soluble vitamins.

[4] Neonates did not present with symptoms suggesting celiac disease or with evidence of pulmonary infection, so Andersen's identification of CF in them was entirely dependent on finding the typical pancreatic lesion at autopsy. These young patients helped persuade her that she was indeed looking at a new disease and suggested to her that the pancreatic lesion might be the underlying defect. A decade later after numerous fetal autopsies, she changed her mind, believing that the pancreas was just one more organ affected by the disease (see next chapter).

[5] The epithelium is a layer of cells that covers body surfaces both internally and externally.

Autopsies in eleven infants or children with celiac syndrome without pancreatic pathology were also reviewed and revealed that these patients died at a later age than those with "cystic fibrosis of the pancreas," and most of them (six of eleven) died due to exacerbations of chronic diarrhea. Patients with the new disease did seem to have a different clinical course compared to those with celiac syndrome and a normal pancreas.

Andersen found that 3% (twenty of six hundred and five) of autopsies in infants or children at Babies Hospital over many years (most performed prior to Andersen's tenure) revealed a pancreatic lesion consistent with this new disease, as she defined it (i.e., more than 90% of the exocrine pancreas was nonfunctional). As some autopsies performed prior to 1935 lacked a description of the pancreas, it was even possible that 3% was an underestimate.

For comparison, a review of Babies Hospital autopsy records revealed that in the two years following the index case, a diagnosis of "cystic fibrosis of the pancreas" was made in ten autopsy reports at Babies Hospital (as noted in the autopsy register). With approximately 70 to 80 autopsies/year at Babies Hospital, about 6% of all autopsies involved infants or children with "cystic fibrosis of the pancreas" during that time. As only half of all deaths at Babies Hospital were then autopsied (e.g., seventy-six of one hundred forty-five in 1935 [7]), the true incidence of this disease in children who died there in the late 1930s is unknown, though it couldn't be any less than Andersen's estimate of 3%, and it might be greater. An unknown disease present in a similar fraction of all pediatric deaths would be startling today; as Andersen wrote: "the incidence of 3.3 per cent seems unusually high for a disease so little known" [3]. She believed that the inclusion of infants and children living with this disease would suggest a disease even more broadly prevalent.

Andersen suggested that therapy for children with "cystic fibrosis of the pancreas" should include, at a minimum, fat-soluble vitamin supplementation and a greater caloric intake than normal. Therapeutic suggestions by a pathologist seemed a bit unusual to clinicians at that time: she didn't care; it was also still the case that no one had yet made a diagnosis of this new disease in a living patient, so it was not clear who would be getting this therapy. Therapeutic suggestions by a female pathologist – and a very junior one, at that – were even less welcome in that era. However her dedication was quickly rewarded: she presented her findings at the 1938 American Pediatric Society/Society for Pediatric Research at Great Barrington, Massachusetts, and received the E. Mead Johnson Award in 1939 [2].[6]

Importantly, discussion which followed the study revealed that recognition of this new disease by clinicians was widespread and immediate [3]. Beryl Paige, as Andersen's supervisor, wrote to Mount Holyoke College's Alumnae Association to spread the word about Andersen's study and her award: "I am sure the alumnae and faculty who know Dr. Andersen will be glad to learn of the recognition given her excellent work" [5].

---

[6]There were two recipients of this award in 1938: Andersen received $300 for her work on CF, while Frederic Gibbs received $500 for his work on epilepsy.

How is it that Andersen's recognition of this pancreatic lesion as a marker of a relatively common disease remained undiscovered by others until 1938? Meticulous expertise in pathology was the first requirement: following her identification of the index case, Andersen examined and reexamined hundreds of autopsy records and material in order to develop her argument. Her experience as an anatomist was critical in this context. However, a superior knowledge of physiology was also required: she needed to frame the argument by considering how this pancreatic lesion led to at least some of the disease symptoms. And finally, Andersen was not the only researcher to pursue investigations of this pancreatic lesion in the 1930s, though her study was the first to provide a firm scientific basis to begin investigations of this new disease. Andersen's study was not a major advance in basic science; rather it was the result of meticulous work in pathology coupled with an understanding of the physiologic implications, and it was knit together with remarkable clinical expertise.

Medical students at the time remembered fondly Andersen's lectures about this new disease, as noted by Freeman Hersey [5] and Jack Docter [8]. Docter was later CF Center Director in Seattle: "I first heard of cystic fibrosis (CF) in 1938, when as a second year medical student at Columbia University, I was privileged to hear Dr. Dorothy Andersen present her description of this new disease" [8]. He added: "It was my further privilege to hear her discuss this disease many times during the next two years, and it made a lasting impression" [8].

However, there was controversy associated with Andersen's 1938 study: at least one of the authors whose patients were included by Andersen (Margaret Harper) and another whose own study appeared just a few months after Andersen's (Charles May) were not disposed to be generous regarding who was first to identify this new disease. Controversy persists about whether the early reports of patients with this new disease (in particular, by Margaret Harper in 1930 [9], Kenneth Blackfan and Burt Wolbach in 1933 [6], Arthur Parmelee in 1935 [10], and Guido Fanconi in 1936 [11], among others) deserve at least as much recognition as Andersen received. However, descriptions of this new disease in these early studies involved fewer patients, with less clinical detail compared to Andersen's study, and Andersen's emphasis on deficiencies in exocrine pancreatic function pointed the way to further investigations of this disease.

Harper voiced a common complaint which focused on Andersen's status as a pathologist: "Andersen's article from the pathological laboratory of the Babies Hospital, New York reported 49 cases culled from various sources; it is written from the pathological standpoint without personal clinical experience of the disease" [12]. Too true in some ways: a clinician might segregate patients with celiac syndrome into those with or without lung disease, while a pathologist might segregate them by the presence or absence of pancreatic disease; and yet the former approach was not terribly helpful as a strategy.[7] Andersen's approach eventually led to wide-

---

[7] Bacterial pneumonia, occasionally with sequelae related to previous episodes, was unfortunately common in the pre-antibiotic era; it is likely that CF patients would then have constituted only a fraction of the patients with celiac syndrome and lung disease.

spread recognition of this new disease – as she had implied a diagnostic strategy involving an assessment of the release of pancreatic enzymes (into the small bowel); attempts to diagnose this new disease based on a clinician's assessment of lung disease symptoms would have been much less successful, as these symptoms were not specific to CF.

It is nevertheless important to recognize the insightful work done by all the early CF investigators, Harper, Blackfan and Wolbach, Parmelee, Fanconi, and others were all focused on the identification of an unknown, potentially life-threatening disease, and they all deserve some share of the credit for its discovery. What is clear in retrospect is that Andersen's 1938 study was the stimulus to a number of subsequent investigations of this new disease, and it served as the beginning of attempts to treat CF. Critics of Andersen's work would have been much less vigorous if the new disease she described was rare; far from it: it turned out to be one of the most common, fatal genetic disorders in the United States and Europe.

Charles May's role as a researcher and critic of Andersen's work deserves further comment. Five years after Blackfan's work at Harvard with Wolbach, Blackfan and May reviewed autopsy results of 35 children who all died before 2 years of age with a pancreatic lesion and a clinical course similar to Andersen's patients [13]. Their study appeared a few months after Andersen's in 1938: "Blackfan's exacting standards had required so many revisions of the paper that he and May were 'beaten to the punch' by Dr. Dorothy Andersen … who is credited with first identifying cystic fibrosis" [14]. Several years after his retirement from Babies Hospital, Rustin McIntosh suggested that Blackfan and May deserved perhaps as much credit as Andersen in recognizing this new disease:

> The scattered and rare case reports published prior to 1938 recognized it only as a concatenation of apparently unrelated lesions of morbid anatomy and gave no hint of its real frequency. By 1938 when Dorothy Andersen in New York and Blackfan and May in Boston first recognized it as a not uncommon disorder of infancy and childhood, amplified its clinical picture and clarified its morphology, the disease was still identifiable with certainty only at post-mortem. [15]

Though McIntosh was the Medical Director of Babies Hospital and thus Andersen's clinical supervisor during the time she made her many contributions to CF care and knowledge, his assessment of her landmark CF study may have been an attempt to appear scrupulously fair.[8]

May later suggested that "the name generally employed for this disease, 'cystic fibrosis of the pancreas,' is misleading [16]" (and instead used the name "fibrosis of the pancreas" [16]). He pointedly avoided recognizing Andersen's 1938 study as a landmark in an extensive monograph on CF he published in 1954 [17]. In a brief review of May's monograph, James Littlewood noted:

---

[8] Perhaps a more accurate assessment is that McIntosh, who had strong ties to Harvard, was not prone to overstating Andersen's accomplishments.

There is an interesting dedication at the beginning [of May's monograph]- "To the practitioners, Margaret Harper of Sydney, Australia and Arthur H Parmelee of Chicago, Illinois who recognised the salient clinical features of patients found to have cystic fibrosis of the pancreas, published the first papers indicating the frequency and importance of the disease, and clearly set it apart from celiac disease against the prevalent practice" … there was no mention of Dorothy Andersen except that "Andersen's original paper should be consulted for the most adequate illustrations of progressive stages in the development of this (pancreatic) lesion". [18]

May's omission of Andersen may reflect in part the frustration he felt working with Blackfan on their 1938 study [13]. In the 1940s May offered criticisms of several of Andersen's recommendations: he suggested that "there is little justification for the use of restricted or special diets in this disorder" [19], a comment which referred to Andersen's recommendation of a low-fat/high-protein diet [20]. He also suggested that "the usefulness of pancreatin is questionable because of its low or uncertain enzyme potency, expense, and the relatively little improvement effected in absorption" [16], another reference to an Andersen recommendation. However, his experience with CF was likely not as extensive as Andersen's.[9]

May joined Babies Hospital in 1957, and though he stayed only a few years, these years overlapped with several of Andersen's last few years. There is nothing to suggest that Andersen was anything but gracious to him, or he to her. Indeed, Andersen remained gracious to all of her critics throughout her career; her responses to criticism always focused on scientific and medical questions only, as she consistently avoided personal conflicts.

Hattie Alexander later wrote about Andersen's 1938 study: "One of the brightest stars in Rusty McIntosh's crown is the contribution of Dorothy Andersen to cystic fibrosis of the pancreas…. This paper is only one of the highlights among the many contributions of Dorothy Andersen to pediatric pathology" [21]. It was Andersen's first significant contribution to medical knowledge, and it was to be the most important work of her career: she had scored her first goal.

Unlike Martha Wollstein, Dorothy Andersen's prestige was unlikely to fade anytime soon: her 1938 study meant that her name would forever be linked to CF. But Andersen had bigger plans: her work on CF was just beginning.

---

[9]Harry Schwachman (Chief of the Division of Clinical Nutrition at the Children's Hospital in Boston) was one of the pioneers of CF care from the 1940s through the 1970s. He suggested that "May's interest in CF was limited because he didn't have a laboratory…and he wrote a textbook [the monograph referred to above] on CF because he wanted to write down his experience before he left the clinic."

References

1. Wright JR Jr, Abrams J. Martha Wollstein of Babies Hospital in New York City (1868-1939)- the first North American pediatric pathologist. Pediatr Dev Pathol. 2018;21(5):437–43.
2. Sicherman B, Green CH. Notable American women: the modern period: a biographical dictionary. Cambridge, MA: The Belknap Press of Harvard University Press; 1980.
3. Andersen DH. Cystic fibrosis of the pancreas and its relation to celiac disease: a clinical and pathologic study. Am J Dis Chil. 1938;56(2):344–99.
4. Trivedi BP. Breath from salt: a deadly genetic disease, a new era in science, and the patients and families who changed medicine forever. BenBella Books, Incorporated; 2020.
5. Dorothy H. Andersen papers. Archives at the Augustus C. Long Health Sciences Library of Columbia University.
6. Blackfan KD, Wolbach SB. Vitamin a deficiency in infants: a clinical and pathological study. J Pediatr. 1933;3(5):679–706.
7. Report of the Dean of the School of Medicine. In: Columbia University bulletin of information. New York: Columbia University; 1931–58.
8. Doershuk CF. Cystic fibrosis in the 20th century: people, events, and progress. Cleveland: AM Publishing Ltd; 2001.
9. Harper MH. Two cases of congenital pancreatic steatorrhea with infantilism. Med J Aust. 1930;2(20):663–4.
10. Parmelee AH. The pathology of steatorrhea. Am J Dis Child. 1935;50(6):1418–28.
11. Fanconi G, Uehlinger E, Knauer C. Das Coeliakiesyndrom bei angeborener zystischer Pankreasfibromatose und Bronchiektasien. Wien Med Wochenschr; 1936.
12. Harper MH. Congenital steatorrhea due to defect of the pancreas. Med J Aust. 1949;1(5):137–41.
13. Blackfan KD, May CD. Inspissation of secretion, dilatation of the ducts and acini, atrophy and fibrosis of the pancreas in infants: a clinical note. J Pediatr. 1938;13(5):627–34.
14. Bergner RK. In memoriam: Charles D. May, M.D. Allergy Asthma Proc. 1993;7(3):230–1.
15. McIntosh R. Progress in cystic fibrosis. Pediatrics. 1965;36(5):673–4.
16. May CD, Lowe CU. Fibrosis of the pancreas in infants and children; an illustrated review of certain clinical features with special emphasis on the pulmonary and cardiac aspects. J Pediatr. 1949;34(6):663–87.
17. May CD. Cystic fibrosis of the pancreas in infants and children, vol. 93. Springfield: Charles C. Thomas; 1954.
18. Littlewood J. A history of cystic fibrosis. 2002. Available from: www.cysticfibrosismedicine.com.
19. May CD, Lowe CU. The treatment of fibrosis of the pancreas in infants and children. Pediatrics. 1948;1(2):159–73.
20. Andersen DH. Celiac syndrome: III. Dietary therapy for congenital pancreatic deficiency. Am J Dis Child. 1945;70(2):100–13.
21. McIntosh R. The McIntosh era at Babies Hospital, 1931–1960: a commemorative volume to honor Rustin McIntosh. Babies Hospital; 1960.

CF Firsts

10

As the first decade of the McIntosh Era at Babies Hospital drew to a close in 1941, several of Rustin McIntosh's goals from 1933 had already been met: Babies Hospital was the major site for Columbia University's Department of Pediatrics as well as the center of an expanded research agenda. Though space constraints continued to limit some of the research efforts, Dorothy Andersen found a lab home[1] on the eighth floor, where she began her numerous CF studies, as well as her investigations into glycogen storage diseases with Howard Mason. The Babies Hospital training program for pediatricians began to attract physicians from all over the United States. During the second decade of the McIntosh Era, Babies Hospital was well-respected and influential in academic pediatrics and was beginning to develop a legacy of research, including therapeutic advances for sick children.

However, World War II was a major disruption for the hospital, as it was for all centers of academic medicine: by the end of 1942, nearly a third (ten of thirty-two) of the faculty were called up to be "in our country's service" [1], and there was no easy way to replace them. As Rustin McIntosh reported:

> Every physically fit male member of the attending staff under the age of thirty-eight years has entered some branch of service, and many in the higher age ranges as well. A number of men on the house staff have gone directly into Army positions after completing the minimum term of hospital training required for a commission; the proportion of those who have been temporarily kept on the "essential" list to meet the pressing need of the hospital organization for experienced personnel has been held down to a bare minimum. [1]

Nearly a third (seven of twenty-two) of the remaining faculty were women [1] (at one point in 1942 the total number of faculty dropped even further to twelve [2]). Babies Hospital was able to absorb some of these losses at the expense of an

---

[1] Andersen's actual home for most of the 1940s was an apartment in Washington Heights just a few blocks from CUMC. For Andersen, the chief virtue of this apartment was its proximity to work, though she also seemed to enjoy the neighborhood's cultural mix: numerous Europeans arrived there in the 1930s, in particular refugees who had escaped from Nazi Germany.

© The Author(s), under exclusive license to Springer Nature Switzerland AG 2022
J. S. Baird, *Dorothy Hansine Andersen*,
https://doi.org/10.1007/978-3-030-87484-1_10

increased workload imposed on those remaining, many of whom were women. In response to the question "How does the war affect your job?", Andersen responded: "doubles it" [3], and this was a common perception. Few complained about the extra work: Andersen's good friend Hilde Bruch lost several siblings and friends to the Nazi holocaust; the Babies Hospital faculty were well aware of the costs in terms of human life associated with the war.

There were numerous questions which demanded Andersen's attention after her 1938 CF study: can a diagnosis of CF be made other than by examining autopsy specimens? What effects do dietary, vitamin, and pancreatic enzyme replacement therapies have on patients with CF? Is there any treatment available for the pulmonary disease associated with CF? Is CF likely to be an infectious, nutritional, or genetic disease? And if genetic, can the inheritance pattern be defined? The work required of Andersen to answer these questions was enormous: she noted in the early 1940s that "2/3 of her time" was spent on "medical research on celiac disease," by which she meant CF. With this research agenda, she moved from autopsy descriptions in 1938 to refinements of medical therapy in a very short time. Her expertise in clinical research seemed to emerge spontaneously, complete with a knowledge of topics as varied as statistics, outpatient care and follow-up, and administrative skills, as well as an understanding of any new, related medical research.

To begin with, a diagnostic strategy seemed like a good bet: assess the output of pancreatic enzymes (amylase, lipase, and trypsin) released into the small bowel to digest food in patients with celiac syndrome. Based on the pathologic findings she noted in 1938, she believed that the secretion of these enzymes would be decreased in the group of celiac syndrome patients who actually had CF.

And indeed, in 1938 she diagnosed "pancreatic insufficiency" in an infant who had symptoms suggesting celiac syndrome: "the duodenal juice was analyzed for enzymes on two occasions; none were found" [4]. She concluded that this patient had a "clinical diagnosis" of CF [4] – and he was the first patient to be diagnosed in vivo (though she was unable to verify that he had anatomic evidence of the pancreatic lesion[2]).

She then verified that pancreatic enzymes obtained by a small tube inserted into the middle third of the duodenum (the first part of the small intestine) were absent or quite low in a cohort of sick children that Andersen identified with "congenital pancreatic deficiency," compared to control (normal) patients or to those with chronic diarrhea and/or severe malnutrition [5]. "Congenital pancreatic deficiency" was the description Andersen used for those patients which she previously considered to have a "clinical diagnosis of CF." Ten of fifteen patients in the cohort of those with low levels of pancreatic enzymes in the duodenum died within a year, and five of these ten underwent autopsy examinations: a diagnosis of CF was verified in all five. This suggested that the absence of pancreatic enzymes in the duodenal secretions confirmed an actual diagnosis of CF.

---

[2] Paul di Sant'Agnese remembered about this patient that he "lived until the age of ten or eleven years, despite the lack of any effective treatment," so a pathologic exam did not occur.

Andersen further noted that trypsin[3] seemed to be preferable to use when attempting to separate patients with CF from the other patients with celiac syndrome [5], and testing for trypsin in duodenal secretions then became the gold standard for CF diagnosis. However, inserting a small tube into a child's duodenum in order to assess the amount of trypsin present in duodenal secretions is not easy to perform; it requires both expertise and specialized equipment. While a medical student at Johns Hopkins, Lewis Gibson had some difficulties performing this procedure, and he wrote to Andersen: "I sometimes encountered considerable difficulty getting a tube through the pylorus and into the duodenum. She replied to my letter and included a drawing of a small brass dumbbell, about the size of two BB shot, which she tied to the end of the duodenal tube." It worked, and Gibson[4] remarked that "I was greatly impressed by the kindness of Dr. Andersen" [6].

A corollary of her work establishing the utility of using pancreatic enzyme analysis for diagnostic purposes was the possible benefit of therapeutic replacement of pancreatic enzymes: she began a vigorous program of diet, vitamins, and pancreatic enzyme replacement therapy in newly diagnosed patients with CF soon after making her first diagnosis. By 1945, Andersen was caring for 38 patients with CF. Her retrospective studies of the clinical course of these CF patients were the first to outline the use of these therapies [4, 7]: she continued to suggest an increased caloric requirement and recommended a low-fat/high-protein diet with supplementary vitamins and pancreatin (a commercial, pancreatic enzyme product available then which was porcine-derived). Andersen suggested that CF patients treated with this regimen had a slightly longer survival compared to historical controls at Babies Hospital, depending on their age and symptoms at the time therapy was initiated.

However, her investigation of the dietary and pancreatic enzyme replacement therapies had to proceed more or less concurrently with investigations of antibiotic therapy: confounding by multiple factors thus limited the interpretation of efficacy for any specific therapy. Andersen made every attempt to isolate each therapy as much as possible, but none of the retrospective data were optimal; Andersen was certainly aware of these limitations, and knew that these limitations contributed to controversy: this was particularly true for her vitamin A deficiency hypothesis.

By the mid-1940s as World War II was winding down, Andersen had some help with her research and clinical work: several recently trained physicians were hired to help with outpatient care for her CF patients, and Andersen began to offer mentorship to those who were interested in research. One of those she mentored was Paul di Sant'Agnese, who coauthored with Andersen the first study on antibiotic therapy in CF [8]. Andersen must have been impressed with his contributions, as he was the first author of this report.

The first antibiotics to be available for use in the United States were the sulfonamides [9], and they were first used in 1935 at Babies Hospital, as previously noted. The sulfonamide antibiotics had "limited usefulness" in CF: 8 of 9 patients with a

---

[3] Trypsin is the pancreatic enzyme which helps digest protein.
[4] Gibson and Robert Cooke later developed the procedure commonly used to obtain sweat in order to test for CF: pilocarpine iontophoresis.

mild respiratory infection responded to therapy compared to only 1 of 19 with evidence of a more severe respiratory infection [8]. In 1943, small quantities of penicillin became available at CUMC, and by 1944 penicillin supplies were "adequate" [8] to permit the use of this new antibiotic in several patients with CF.[5] The authors investigated both intramuscular and aerosolized penicillin (not intravascular) for staphylococcal pneumonia: only one of five patients treated with intramuscular penicillin "had a satisfactory response",[6] while "excellent success" was noted in five of ten patients treated with aerosolized penicillin [8]. As a result, di Sant'Agnese and Andersen suggested using aerosolized penicillin alone or in combination with intramuscular penicillin for severe respiratory infections in CF [8]. They also suggested that antibiotics were responsible for at least some improvement in CF survival. Their investigation of aerosolized penicillin was performed with the expertise and assistance of Alvan Barach – an extraordinarily interesting CUMC physician with extensive experience as an innovator in the care of lung disease in adults[7] – who provided the aerosol apparatus for use in the CF investigations (Fig. 10.1).[8]

Also in 1946, Andersen collaborated with Richard Hodges on the first report to affirm that CF is a genetic disease which behaves in a recessive manner:[9] they reported the incidence of CF in siblings of CF patients at Babies Hospital and in the medical literature and also investigated family pedigrees of 20 CF patients at Babies Hospital [10]. They noted a disease incidence in siblings of approximately 25%, as well as frequent evidence of CF "in several branches of the family tree." This study "is the first clear statement, backed by clinical evidence, that CF is inherited in a Mendelian recessive manner" [11].

It is notable that a decade later Andersen wavered a bit:[10] "The present general opinion that the disease is a recessive doesn't seem to me right, first, because of the low incidence of consanguinity- we had 2 instances in 400 cases, about the normal

---

[5]The university's source of penicillin was likely the federal government's Office of Scientific Research and Development, though Hattie Alexander's collaborator Geoffrey Rake was by then working at the Squibb Corporation helping to develop its rapidly growing capacity to produce penicillin, and he may also have played some role in its availability. Credit to di Sant'Agnese for getting "several vials of the precious drug" from a "uniformed colonel" at CUMC has also been suggested, though di Sant'Agnese and Andersen themselves also credited Alvan Barach for obtaining a supply of the antibiotic. An exact attribution for the source of all the penicillin used in this study is likely impossible.

[6]Penicillin therapy was limited by drug supply; in addition, several of these patients had at least short-term improvement, followed by deterioration with the emergence of drug-resistant strains of bacteria.

[7]Barach helped develop or assist in the development of oxygen tents and oxygen therapy, helium oxygen mixtures for airway obstruction, aerosol delivery of bronchodilators and other drugs, and the cough assist device for those unable to cough effectively.

[8]Aerosolized antibiotic therapy for CF would emerge again in the second half of the twentieth century as an important therapeutic option to help suppress the growth of *Pseudomonas* bacteria.

[9]A recessive genetic disease is expressed when the gene contributed by each parent is abnormal, while a dominant genetic disease is expressed when the gene – or allele – contributed by only one parent is abnormal.

[10]From a 1956 letter to Harry Schwachman.

Fig. 10.1 In 1926, a year after helping to develop this technology, Alvan Barach posed in one of his oxygen tents. (In the public domain)

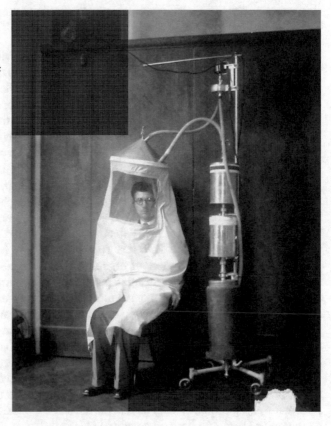

rate, and second, because of the high carrier rate of genes in the general population required" [3]. She had become convinced that something was a bit off in the statistics, as, in theory, an increase in consanguinity should be associated with an increased incidence of autosomal recessive disorders. She could not then know that a multitude of various CF allelic defects might be associated with dissimilar disease manifestations; indeed, the clinical effect of a combination of any two defective, but different, alleles might be difficult to predict.

Andersen and Hodges also pondered the underlying defect of CF in their 1946 study: as the pancreatic lesion was key to her recognition of the disease in 1938 and seemed to be the earliest recognizable abnormality to develop in her patients, she looked for evidence that this was the underlying problem. Back in 1938, she had suggested that the pancreatic lesion may develop during fetal life and suggested that this could be a key to understanding the disease. However by 1946, Andersen had a slightly different understanding:

> The lesion in the pancreas is not a malformation in the true sense of the word but appears in the latter part of pregnancy. It probably results from an abnormality of the acinar secretion. A comparable disturbance is also found in the liver, the gallbladder and the intestines and

possibly in other glands… the pulmonary lesion begins after birth and is primarily the result of nutritional deficiency. [10]

This nutritional deficiency was, Andersen then believed, vitamin A deficiency. As Beryl Paige had by then reviewed numerous fetal autopsies at Babies Hospital without finding any evidence of a well-developed pancreatic lesion early in fetal life, Andersen and Hodges suggested that the pancreatic abnormality was progressive over time, that it was not the underlying defect of CF, and that the clinical manifestations she had described affecting the pancreas, the liver, and the intestines of children with CF all reflected some basic, underlying defect in glandular secretion; this was a recurring theme for Andersen. She did not believe that the disease reflected an isolated defect in, for example, mucous glands alone. Rather the disease involved many different exocrine (not endocrine) glands, including perhaps those responsible for the production of saliva, tears, wax, and sweat, in addition to mucous.

Speculation about the primary defect in CF led other researchers to a different conclusion: in 1944 Sidney Farber at Harvard noted the important role in CF of thick, sticky mucus in a variety of organs [12] and suggested the primary defect involved mucous glands. He was also convinced that vitamin A deficiency in this disease was not a primary problem leading to lung disease, but a result of malabsorption. As a result, "an on-going conflict between Harvard and Columbia about the nature of the disease" [6] emerged: Farber suggested that the disease be renamed mucoviscidosis. Attribution of the principal defect in CF to mucus glands seemed a little far-fetched to Andersen, and in 1950 she commented: "I think that the use of this word [mucoviscidosis] has the semantic ill effect of giving one the illusion that the basic causation of the disease is known. It is possible but not proved that the pancreatic and pulmonary lesions rest on the same mechanism, and until proof is forthcoming I prefer to keep an open mind" [13].[11]

While both CF and vitamin A deficiency involve disturbances of epithelial cells including some of their associated glands, what Andersen – as well as Farber and all of the early CF researchers – did not then know was that CF is an epithelial cell channelopathy;[12] the channel responsible for CF is known as the CF transmembrane conductance regulator, or CFTR. It is responsible for regulating the movement of ions across epithelial cell membranes, and it was first described by Paul Quinton in 1983 [14]. The gene responsible for making the protein which constitutes the CFTR

---

[11] It is ironic that one of the first investigators to suggest the importance of vitamin A deficiency in infants with pulmonary disease was Kenneth Blackfan at Harvard and even more ironic that Charles May, who worked with Blackfan, favored a related name for this new disease: fibrosis of the pancreas. Though Andersen occasionally used a slight variant of the name she originally chose for this disease during the first decade following her initial study (fibrocystic disease of the pancreas), in the end, the shortened name she used late in her career – cystic fibrosis – was gradually adopted. It is also ironic that in 1950 she was also working on her study of heat prostration in CF: as will be seen in a later chapter, this study helped to establish a new paradigm in CF, confirming the involvement of non-mucous secreting glands in the disease.

[12] A channelopathy is an abnormality in an ion channel in the membranes of cells (commonly the defect involves a protein).

channel is located on chromosome seven; this gene was discovered by a team led by Lap-Chee Tsui in 1989 [15]. Different mutations of this gene – over 2000 were described prior to 2021 – confer some of the differences in the severity of CF based on their effects on the structure and function of the CFTR protein, as well as on the protein's ability to move to its correct position and function in an epithelial cell. As CF is a recessive genetic disorder, abnormal genes from both parents are essential to produce the disease, and the mutations may not be identical, compounding the complexity.

The effects of a CFTR channelopathy include abnormal transport of ions and water, leading potentially to a dehydrated surface layer sitting atop epithelial cells. However, there are also organ-specific effects: in the pancreas, abnormal CFTR is associated with deficient bicarbonate ion transport which may lead to the disruption of multiple intracellular processes [16], while in airways, abnormal CFTR is associated with thickened airway secretions related to infection and inflammation. Interestingly, it does not appear that CFTR mediates the production or release of mucus in airways directly [17].

However, all this only became known decades later. By then, interest in a better name for CF had faded. As di Sant'Agnese wrote years later:

> Cystic fibrosis, therefore, is not a disease of the pancreas but one in which this organ is frequently but not necessarily involved. The name commonly given this generalized disorder is a misnomer; however, it is accepted by tradition and it brings to mind a known symptom complex. Therefore, until the etiology of this condition is further clarified and a more precise term found, the name cystic fibrosis of the pancreas can be used with the full realization of its limitations. [18]

CF is characterized by the abnormal movement of ions and water across epithelial cell membranes leading to alterations which affect most epithelial surfaces, though the underlying defect is not specifically a gland abnormality[13] (so Andersen was not quite correct). In addition, lung disease is not produced by the same processes which are responsible for the pancreatic lesion, as there are organ-specific effects (so that Farber was not correct either). But enough quibbling: CF is a complicated disease involving multiple organ systems as a result of a defective cell membrane channel. How common is it?

Based on population data in New York City in the 1940s, Andersen and Hodges suggested an incidence for CF of 1.7 to 1.8 per thousand live births in New York City, but this was an overestimate: the actual incidence may only be as high as 0.3 to 0.5 per thousand live births in northern European populations. Diagnostic criteria have changed since the 1940s, and it is at least possible that the use of duodenal enzyme assays to diagnose CF was associated with false positive results (e.g., testing could, in theory, have been positive for some patients with chronic pancreatitis). Nevertheless, CF is still considered a common genetic disease, at least in northern European populations.

---

[13] It is, of course, true that cells which make up the sweat glands do contain CFTR and that sweat testing is a reliable method of diagnosing CF (see Chap. 13).

Andersen reviewed her first decade of clinical experience at Babies Hospital with CF [19] and concluded: "Early diagnosis and therapy lead to an improved prognosis, and may result in freedom from respiratory infection, at least for the span of years over which observation has been possible." As treatment for these patients included vitamin supplementation and nutritional support, this led her to conclude that "There is strong presumptive evidence that it [lung infection] is due to a specific nutritional deficiency" [20]. She clung to the vitamin A deficiency hypothesis for several reasons which are less convincing several decades later: early supplementation with vitamin A seemed to be associated with a cohort of Andersen's CF patients who had delayed onset of lung disease, and a delay in dietary and vitamin therapy in other patients seemed to be associated with acquisition of lung disease at a younger age. However, the principal organs affected by vitamin A deficiency are known to be the eyes and skin, and variability in CF lung disease severity may be associated with a variety of (non-CFTR related) genetic and environmental factors- or disease modifiers- which are still being investigated.

Though it took a great deal of planning and extra work on Andersen's part, Andersen's last major investigation in the 1940s involved her vitamin A deficiency hypothesis: could vitamin A deficiency in utero lead to CF in an animal model? Though she originally suspected that vitamin A deficiency secondary to fat malabsorption was responsible only for CF-associated lung disease, she had also become concerned that some of the variability in the severity and timing of CF disease might depend on the severity and timing of fetal exposure to vitamin A deficiency. Earlier in the 1930s, she had worked in an animal lab (mainly with rats) to pursue her studies on female reproduction, and some of the skills she learned then were adapted to this new investigation. Andersen published her results in 1949 and showed that experimental maternal vitamin A deficiency in rats was not associated with CF in their offspring [21], though it was frequently associated with congenital diaphragmatic hernia.

By the 1950s, Andersen no longer believed that vitamin A deficiency was a significant underlying cause of lung disease in CF:

> Although most observers, including the author, no longer regard the bronchitis as the direct result of deficiency of vitamin A or other nutritional factors, good nutrition prior to severe infection greatly increases resistance in these children. [22]

It was clear by the late 1940s that an improvement in survival for patients with CF had occurred. One of Andersen's case reports [8] offered an example: an infant girl had failure to thrive and large, foul-smelling stools since birth. Andersen noted that she also had frequent upper respiratory tract infections beginning at 2 months of age. At 7 months of age, she was treated with penicillin for "pneumonia followed by a pulmonary abscess," and she was diagnosed with CF at 11 months of age. She then began a low-fat/high-protein diet with pancreatic enzyme replacement and vitamins. At 12 and 15 months of age, she was again treated with penicillin for pneumonia. At 23 months of age, she had gained weight and was well at a follow-up visit

[8]. Andersen had suggested in 1938 that young infants with CF and failure to thrive, chronic cough, and pulmonary infections did not survive for long. However, by the end of the 1940s, some infants who received CF treatment as Andersen recommended – focused on nutrition, pancreatic enzyme replacement, and antibiotics for pulmonary infection – did survive into childhood.

In 1948, a decade after her landmark 1938 CF study and following the publication of her many "CF firsts," Andersen was promoted to one of the lower rungs on the academic career ladder: assistant professor (of pathology). While it is difficult to be precise about the appropriate time course of academic promotions in response to academic accomplishments, this suggests a delay in advancement.

It didn't seem to bother her.

References

1. Annual report of the Babies Hospital of the City of New York. New York: The Babies Hospital of the City of New York; 1889–1942.
2. Presbyterian Hospital. Annual report of the Presbyterian Hospital in the City of New York. New York: The Presbyterian Hospital in the City of New York; 1939-64.
3. Dorothy H. Andersen papers. Archives at the Augustus C. Long Health Sciences Library of Columbia University.
4. Andersen DH. Cystic fibrosis of the pancreas, vitamin A deficiency, and bronchiectasis. J Pediatr. 1939;15(6):763–71.
5. Andersen DH. Pancreatic enzymes in the duodenal juice in the celiac syndrome. Am J Dis Child. 1942;63(4):643–58.
6. Doershuk CF. Cystic fibrosis in the 20th century: people, events, and progress. Cleveland: AM Publishing Ltd; 2001.
7. Andersen DH. Celiac syndrome: III. Dietary therapy for congenital pancreatic deficiency. Am J Dis Child. 1945;70(2):100–13.
8. Di Sant'Agnese PA, Andersen DH. Celiac syndrome; chemotherapy in infections of the respiratory tract associated with cystic fibrosis of the pancreas; observations with penicillin and drugs of the sulfonamide group, with special reference to penicillin aerosol. Am J Dis Child. 1946;72:17–61.
9. Carithers HA. The first use of an antibiotic in America. Am J Dis Child. 1974;128(2):207–11.
10. Andersen DH, Hodges RG. Celiac syndrome; genetics of cystic fibrosis of the pancreas, with a consideration of etiology. Am J Dis Child. 1946;72:62–80.
11. Littlewood J. A history of cystic fibrosis. 2002. Available from: www.cysticfibrosismedicine.com.
12. Farber S. Pancreatic function and disease in early life. V. Pathologic changes associated with pancreatic insufficiency in early life. Arch Pathol. 1944;37:238–50.
13. Schwachman H, Patterson P, Farber S. Significance of altered viscosity of duodenal content in pancreatic fibrosis (mucoviscidosis). AMA Am J Dis Child. 1950;80(5):864–5.
14. Quinton PM. Chloride impermeability in cystic fibrosis. Nature. 1983;301(5899):421–2.
15. Kerem B, et al. Identification of the cystic fibrosis gene: genetic analysis. Science. 1989;245(4922):1073–80.
16. Madácsy T, Pallagi P, Maleth J. Cystic fibrosis of the pancreas: the role of CFTR channel in the regulation of intracellular $Ca(2+)$ signaling and mitochondrial function in the exocrine pancreas. Front Physiol. 2018;9:1585.
17. Kreda SM, Davis CW, Rose MC. CFTR, mucins, and mucus obstruction in cystic fibrosis. Cold Spring Harb Perspect Med. 2012;2(9):a009589.
18. Di Sant'Agnese PA. Introduction to the study of cystic fibrosis of the pancreas: muscoviscidosis, fibrocystic disease of the pancreas. Ann N Y Acad Sci. 1962;93(12):489–99.

19. Andersen DH. Therapy and prognosis of fibrocystic disease of the pancreas. Pediatrics. 1949;3(4):406–17.
20. Andersen DH. The present diagnosis and therapy of cystic fibrosis of the pancreas. Proc R Soc Med. 1949;42(1):25–32.
21. Andersen DH. Effect of diet during pregnancy upon the incidence of congenital hereditary diaphragmatic hernia in the rat; failure to produce cystic fibrosis of the pancreas by maternal vitamin A deficiency. Am J Pathol. 1949;25(1):163–85.
22. Andersen DH. Cystic fibrosis of the pancreas. J Chronic Dis. 1958;7(1):58–90.

"To Dr. Andersen Who Has Pulled Me Through Many a Tough Year"

11

By the time of her promotion to assistant professor, Dorothy Andersen's CF clinic at Babies Hospital had diagnosed one hundred and seven patients with CF; thirty-two of these patients had died, most before 1944 [1]. As news of Andersen's work spread both in the scientific and lay press, patients and families came from great distances to consult with her about a possible diagnosis of CF for their children [2]. They came with both dread and hope and to learn all they could about this frightening disease. Their arrival helped turn Babies Hospital into one of the most important medical centers for CF care during the McIntosh Era:

> As the news spread that there was a doctor at Babies Hospital who had found a way of diagnosing pancreatic insufficiency, suspected cases began to be referred from other hospitals all over the city. A Celiac Clinic was established on the fourth floor of the Vanderbilt Clinic. It met every Thursday morning, with Dr. Andersen … [3]

While many of the consultations for possible CF began in Dr. Andersen's office at Babies Hospital outside of clinic hours, patients diagnosed with CF were then followed up in the outpatient clinic with the assistance of several recently-trained pediatricians over the years: Richard Hodges, Paul di Sant'Agnese, Agnes Wilson, and Carolyn Denning, among others. A request to see a new patient in 1950 illustrates the way many of these consultations were handled, as reported by Dr. Milton Graub, the parent of this patient and also a pediatrician:

> Our son Lee was 2 years old and had been coughing since birth, in addition to having abnormal stools. We had visited local pediatricians and the consultants at the Philadelphia Children's Hospital but I was not satisfied with the diagnosis… I searched the literature and realized that Lee might have a fatal and rare disease, Cystic Fibrosis of the Pancreas… I was so distraught I called Dr. Andersen, on a Sunday morning and found her in her laboratory office. She listened to the medical history of my son and saw him the next day. These were the pre-sweat test days. The diagnosis was much more difficult and was made, primarily on clinical findings plus analysis of duodenal secretions. These were done and the diagnosis of

© The Author(s), under exclusive license to Springer Nature Switzerland AG 2022
J. S. Baird, *Dorothy Hansine Andersen*,
https://doi.org/10.1007/978-3-030-87484-1_11

cystic fibrosis of the pancreas was established. Since Dr. Andersen was a pathologist, she referred Lee for further clinical care to Dr. Paul di Sant'Agnese. He was a pediatric specialist and a delight. [4]

Dr. Graub was one of the first members of the Board of Trustees of the National CF Research Foundation (NCFRF) and served as the NCFRF President in 1964.

In 1953, Doris Tulcin's infant daughter was also evaluated by Dr. Andersen at Babies Hospital:

We called to the Babies Hospital to make an appointment with Dr. Anderson [sic], an amazing woman who was actually a Ph.D. and not an MD. She had discovered this disease back in 1938. She brilliantly started to put some interesting symptoms together. She noticed that babies were dying of heat prostration and salt loss during a very hot summer in New York. [5]

Years later this infant's mother – Doris Tulcin – became involved in the birth and growth of the NCFRF, and in 1976 she also served as NCFRF President.

Andersen's fame as a researcher led some to believe she was not a medical doctor. As pathologists do not generally participate in clinical care, this may have added to the confusion. However, as previously noted, Andersen was both a medical doctor and the recipient of a doctorate degree, and the clinical skills she developed during her surgery internship were sharpened by her research.

The consultation with Tulcin's daughter led to a diagnosis:

Dr. Andersen diagnosed her with CF. This diagnosis was made through the standard duodenal drainage procedure …. The diagnosis was a tremendous blow to our family. Dr. Andersen told us that there was not a great future for our daughter and possibly she might have a year to live. We were very heartbroken parents…. We were then directed to a wonderful pediatrician at Babies Hospital, Dr. Agnes Wilson, who worked with us to get this child on the right road. [4]

Tulcin also had praise for Carolyn Denning, who cared for her daughter a decade later. Parents and family frequently shared positive experiences about many of the physicians providing care for infants and children with CF at Babies Hospital during the McIntosh Era.

In spite of Andersen's appointment as a pathologist, her role as a clinician was vital, as it was Andersen's evaluation which led to a diagnosis of CF. Though in later years Andersen was criticized because "she lacked the ability to take care of the children that were referred to her for care" [6], this was not true: she was appointed Assistant Attending Pediatrician at Babies Hospital in 1945 [7] in addition to her position as Assistant Pathologist. In other words, Rustin McIntosh – as well as Columbia University – recognized her clinical skills: she had completed an internship in surgery, she was frequently called upon to serve as a pediatric ward attending physician at Babies Hospital, and she had by then engaged in a decade's worth of research on CF. It is true that the burden of an ever-expanding population of CF patients, coupled with her duties as a pathologist, as well as her numerous research projects, greatly limited her clinical time: but she was a clinician as well as a pathologist, with all the appropriate knowledge, skill, and instincts needed for good patient care. She also had more than empathy:[1] she was sympathetic to her patients and their pitiable plight.

Andersen's sympathetic nature is reflected in the sentiments expressed by patients and their families. Correspondence in the CUMC Archives [2] include examples of their bond with Andersen, including this letter from a parent who had already lost a child to CF: "You are an extra parent to these children and you give them love and sympathy that is quite separate from your intellectual gifts." This parent had another child that she strongly suspected also had CF: "I [would] like for you to see … [her other child] once in a while- always." One of her CF patients wrote to Andersen: "I had wanted to tell you of my progress for which you are so largely responsible… With my deep affection and true appreciation always." A valentine card from another patient read: "To Dr. Andersen who has pulled me through many a tough year". Andersen commented in a 1955 article in the Ladies Home Journal that "You can't work with these children [with CF] and not come to think of them as yours in some way" [8]. Andersen was greatly respected and loved by her CF patients and their families, and she returned that affection.

Though survival for patients with CF improved during the first few decades following Andersen's 1938 study, the median survival in 1957 was still estimated to be only 5 years of age [4]. Death prior to adulthood in the mid-1950s was unfortunately common for CF patients and often preceded by multiple hospitalizations for exacerbations of their pulmonary disease. However, patients and families remained devoted to someone who could give them information, even if it was uncomfortable information, as long as they were also offered some kind of hope: Andersen and her colleagues fulfilled that role. The courage required of patients and their families in this setting, no less than of the medical team providing the care, was enormous.

Much of the information Andersen supplied was cutting edge, at least for that era. It is important to remember the context: mechanical ventilation was mostly unknown, antibiotics were still being developed and adapted to clinical use, and the efficacy of many medical therapies was unknown, particularly in children. Several examples of the medical advice Andersen dispensed to CF families in her correspondence (from the CUMC Archives [2]) follow:

- In response to a question about aerosol delivery of medications in a patient living in California: "The special apparatus and preparations to be used seem to differ on the East and West coasts. I do not know the Bird breather. In general, there are several pumps which do very well for the use of antibiotics by aerosol. The one which we find satisfactory is the Aero-Mist.[2]"

---

[1] Empathy is to some extent a learned response to the suffering of others, in which we understand and share someone else's emotions, while sympathy is a response – like pity – that seems to be hardwired into many people. As James Joyce noted: "Pity is the feeling which arrests the mind in the presence of whatsoever is grave and constant in human sufferings and unites it with the human sufferer."

[2] A nebulization device used to deliver medication as a mist.

- In response to a question about medications: "The vitamin A should be adequate. I have not been impressed with Monitan.[3]"
- In response to a question about therapy with animal cells: "I would certainly say that no injection with a preparation of animal cells is known which will benefit a child with CF."
- In response to a parent's concern about worsening pulmonary function in a patient in California: "I have no suggestions as to treatment for P____. It is better for doctors on the spot to give advice, than for me at this distance, anyway."

There were also nearly continuous requests for consultations; she gracefully answered a parental request from Australia inquiring whether they should bring their child to the United States to see her: "If you or your doctor feel the need of help from a doctor with considerable experience with cystic fibrosis, you can find one in Australia, without the trouble and expense of a trip here" [2]. She recommended Charlotte Anderson at the University of Melbourne (Anderson later achieved fame in Australia and Britain as a clinician and researcher in CF as well as in celiac disease [9]). Though Andersen did indeed provide consultations to hundreds of patients, she often referred consults to other, trusted physicians. She did not pursue consultations; rather they pursued her.

It was inevitable with the number of patients affected by CF that local, regional, national, and eventually international groups dedicated to CF patients' and their parents' or family's concerns would develop: providing updated medical information was a primary goal, but so was consideration of funding research, setting research priorities, and pursuit of an ultimate cure. Andersen was involved with the development of several of these groups, and some of her contributions in this context will be reviewed in a later chapter. In any case, her support of these early parent groups was clear:

> I'm glad to hear that the San Diego Cystic Fibrosis Group is so active. The New York Group is also very active and has become a sort of club, with a real objective and a good sociable time achieving it. [2]

In spite of Andersen's clinical skills and research in CF, her support of CF patients and families, and her support of the emerging groups or clubs which began to coalesce around CF families, Andersen had occasional critics. To be fair, her character and appearance may not have appealed to everyone: she smoked almost incessantly in the 1950s, as remembered by parents of children with CF [4], and may even have occasionally dropped ashes onto the shoulders of her white lab coat [10]. Her approach to dress and grooming suggested that she was less concerned with her outward appearance than others were, though she was not disheveled. Andersen's candor and honesty with patients and their families may have seemed brutal to some parents: hearing from her that an infant or child with CF was unlikely

---

[3]A solution of polysorbate 80; it was used as an aid to fat digestion in the 1950s, though without real evidence of efficacy, and is not currently recommended.

to survive into adulthood was an overwhelming event, and it is possible that some parents never forgave her for that.

However Andersen's approach as a physician with expertise in CF was not didactic or authoritarian; rather she seems to have been gently persuasive – with almost everyone. Her personality and disposition appeared constant throughout her career: calm, taciturn, and self-deprecatory; she did not complain much. And dishonesty was not an approach she could ever countenance.

Early in 1949 Andersen was asked to provide a photo of herself for Mount Holyoke College, and her reply – in her typical, spidery handwriting – was one of the few complaints she made in writing, though it also reflected her own lack of pretensions and her self-deprecatory nature:

> I am in the unusual position for me of having recently had photos taken… Today it [the glossy print] arrived but is touched up beyond recognition… The photographer had the poor judgement to remodel me… [2]

She refused to use a retouched photo, as she was scrupulously honest even about her own appearance; her fame and renown did not alter her self-regard or make her cocky or vain. Honesty and candor were essential components of her personality, while her demeanor was characterized by modesty and an unassuming nature (Fig. 11.1).

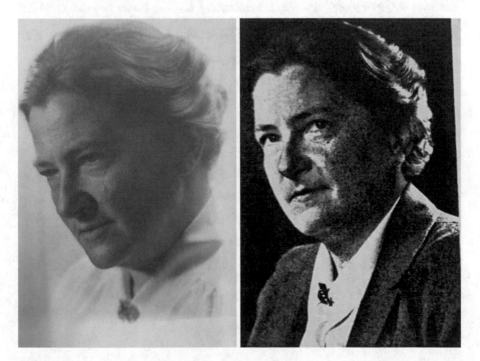

Fig. 11.1 Andersen in 1948: on the left is the retouched photo, and on the right the photo she submitted to Mount Holyoke College. (Courtesy of Archives & Special Collections, Health Sciences Library, Columbia University)

By the end of her first decade at Babies Hospital, she was widely recognized by CF patients and families for her clinical care as well as for the care and concern she lavished upon patients and families. She was a valued member of the Babies Hospital faculty, active in both pediatrics and pathology.

It is possible that she was even a bit too valuable.

References

1. Di Sant'Agnese PA, Andersen DH. Celiac syndrome; chemotherapy in infections of the respiratory tract associated with cystic fibrosis of the pancreas; observations with penicillin and drugs of the sulfonamide group, with special reference to penicillin aerosol. Am J Dis Child. 1946;72:17–61.
2. Dorothy H. Andersen papers. Archives at the Augustus C. Long Health Sciences Library of Columbia University.
3. Machol L. Ahead of her time: a biography of Dorothy H. Andersen, M.D.
4. Doershuk CF. Cystic fibrosis in the 20th century: people, events, and progress. Cleveland: AM Publishing Ltd; 2001.
5. Tulcin DF. Memoirs of a monarch. New York: iUniverse, Inc; 2008.
6. Cystic fibrosis witness seminar by the Wellcome Trust for the History of Medicine. London: The Trustee of the Wellcome Trust, UCL; 2002.
7. Presbyterian Hospital. Annual report of the Presbyterian Hospital in the City of New York. New York: The Presbyterian Hospital in the City of New York; 1939-64.
8. Rustin McIntosh papers. Archives at the Augustus C. Long Health Sciences Library of Columbia University.
9. Walker-Smith J. Obituary of Charlotte Anderson. J Pediatr Gastroenterol Nutr. 2002;35(4):589–90.
10. Damrosch DS. Dorothy Hansine Andersen. J Pediatr. 1964;65:477–9.

McIntosh, Pediatric Pathology, and Columbia University

12

On April 19, 1949, Rustin McIntosh submitted his resignation as Reuben Carpentier professor and Chair of Pediatrics at Columbia University to Columbia University President Dwight D. Eisenhower.

Plans by hospital and medical school administrators to move the pediatric pathology labs from the eighth floor of Babies Hospital to another building on the medical school campus had been developed over the previous year (in part to accommodate the inclusion of the New York Orthopaedic Hospital into CUMC [1]; this hospital was eventually folded into CUMC in 1950). McIntosh realized that this plan would remove not just the resources immediately available in these labs, but also the pathologists: Dorothy Andersen would no longer have a continuous presence at Babies Hospital.

Though moving pediatric pathology labs to free up space at Babies Hospital was something he had also considered early in his tenure, he had since become convinced of Andersen's value; her clinical research in CF included several of the more important contributions to medicine made at Babies Hospital during the McIntosh Era, and moving her to an off-site location would likely limit her research agenda greatly. Babies Hospital was by then one of the most important centers for CF care, and Andersen was critical to that mission.

McIntosh was initially careful to frame his argument against this move in general terms, including insights into his ideas about the mission of Babies Hospital specifically and of academic pediatrics generally. He first explored the importance of pathology to the practice of pediatrics, concluding that:

> The pathologist is forever puzzling over the nature of disease. So does the clinician, but his angle of approach is different. When the two get together, the chances of progress are enhanced. New ideas, fresh attacks, are as apt to be generated in a casual chat as in a scheduled consultation- in fact, probably more so. [1]

The clarity of McIntosh's arguments was then brought to an exploration of practical costs and benefits:

© The Author(s), under exclusive license to Springer Nature Switzerland AG 2022
J. S. Baird, *Dorothy Hansine Andersen*,
https://doi.org/10.1007/978-3-030-87484-1_12

What would be gained if pediatric pathology were moved to the medical school building on 168th Street? Dr. Harry P. Smith, Professor of Pathology, believes that the teaching of pathology to medical students would be improved, and that the opportunities for the education of his own staff in pathology would be enhanced… The claim rests on the assumption that a pediatric pathologist working in the laboratories of the medical school, could carry on at the same high level of productivity and efficiency as now obtains in the pathological laboratory at Babies Hospital. The assertion ignores the sterilizing effect of physical separation from the significant clinical contact. [1]

He noted that a round trip walking from Babies Hospital wards to the CUMC pathology laboratories would take at least 12 minutes (it is easy to envision him carefully timing this journey several times with a stopwatch), and he believed that this would likely curtail contact between pathologist and pediatrician. He went on to consider the consequences:

What, on the other hand, would be lost if pediatric pathology were moved to the medical school building? In the first place, there would be a serious reduction in the research activity of the type which depends upon close cooperation between the pediatrician and the pathologist. This type of work has been an important asset to the Department of Pediatrics for many years. Let me cite as an example the investigations carried out by Dr. Dorothy Andersen and her colleagues in the field of nutritional disorders. Her studies, beginning with an anatomical discovery around 1936, have now been extended to encompass active investigations carried on in living patients on the wards, in clinic and in the private offices. For her work she has received the Mead Johnson award and the Borden award of the American Academy of Pediatrics, both coveted honors of high distinction. Since 1940 her research activities have been supported by the Commonwealth Fund to a total of more than $47,000[1] up to July 1, 1949. Not long ago she received an unsolicited visit from a representative of the John and Mary Markle Foundation, who said that Mr. Whitney had been impressed by the help Dr. Andersen had contributed to the care of one of his grandchildren. When asked whether she needed any additional financial support for her work, Dr. Andersen mentioned a project which would require $5000 a year for a two year period. She was told that it would be prudent on her part to revise her estimate upward. [1]

It is likely that McIntosh continued to frame the argument at meetings mostly in general terms, by suggesting that the "handful of really good pediatric pathologists in this country today … without a single exception, now work in laboratories located in pediatric hospitals" [1]. The logic of this situation reflected the underlying assumption that "really good pediatric pathologists" would be unwilling to work elsewhere. And both Andersen and Paige, in McIntosh's estimation, belonged to that elite group.

It appears, however, that some of the Babies Hospital faculty understood the situation to be a simple power struggle over Dorothy Andersen, as suggested by Richard Day years later:

Pathology at Babies Hospital had been under Martha Wollstein; she was succeeded by Beryl Paige and Dorothy Andersen. Dorothy made this specialty important to both the advancement of knowledge, and by virtue of the laboratory being near the wards, the education of the interns and the staff. Willard Rappleye, Dean at the P&S Medical Center,

---

[1] It is worth noting that 1949 dollars are equivalent to about ten times that amount 70 years later.

> perhaps impressed by her work on cystic fibrosis of the pancreas, wanted to have her and
> her laboratory moved to a spot far from the wards of Babies. Rusty struggled against this
> idea to the point of resigning. [2]

While it is difficult to envision how removing Andersen from Babies Hospital could advance the Dean's academic goals, it is likely that a reorganized and more centralized Department of Pathology would have had the potential to better advance its own academic mission. However, McIntosh was persistent in his argument: pediatric pathologists on site are more likely to be associated with improved pediatric care.

It is notable that Millicent Carey McIntosh, McIntosh's wife, was then the Dean of Barnard College at Columbia University (she eventually was named the first President of Barnard College in 1952): the McIntosh family was deeply embedded in Columbia University. More importantly, respect for McIntosh was widespread: support for his position poured into Columbia University from national and international sources after news of his resignation spread. In spite of a plea from the Dean of Columbia University's College of Physicians and Surgeons (Rappleye), to withdraw his resignation, McIntosh refused. The controversy surrounding the proposed move had been percolating between the Planning Committee of the Medical Board, the trustees of Presbyterian Hospital, the Committee on Administration of the Faculty of Medicine, the Dean of the medical school, and McIntosh – for nearly a year.

Following McIntosh's resignation, there were almost immediate repercussions within Babies Hospital itself:

> At that juncture Rusty called a meeting of his senior staff at which he outlined the facts. He
> concluded with something of a bombshell. He had, he said, told the trustees that an order
> from them to comply was tantamount to asking for his resignation. There was a quaver in
> his voice which defined the depth of his emotion. After a stunned silence, someone
> announced that he would follow Rusty with his own resignation, and he was followed by a
> virtually unanimous declaration of the same intent. [1]

McIntosh must have spoken to Andersen about this situation (no doubt to ensure that she wished to remain at Babies Hospital), though no evidence of this conversation exists. In turn, Andersen must have reassured him that she remained committed to Babies Hospital: by then there were more than a hundred CF patients in the clinic, and she was pursuing several clinical research projects in which access to Babies Hospital facilities and patients was vital (one of these was the CF heat prostration study which she published in 1951). Her lack of interest in public disagreements led her to remain quiet throughout this episode, but she must have been grateful to McIntosh for his leadership.

Did she have any misgivings? It is worth noting that after her return from Europe toward the end of 1948, Andersen was congratulated by Dean Rappleye for the Borden Award: "This is a splendid recognition of the things you are doing and we are pleased to know of that acknowledgement of your work." Andersen responded in January 1949: "It was most thoughtful of you to write such a gracious note. The most pleasant part of the Borden Award has been the expression of appreciation of the home team" [3]. Significantly, she saved his letter and her response,[2] suggesting that she may have believed this interchange to be important. Perhaps she felt that it was linked to McIntosh's resignation in some way, similar to what Richard Day suggested: "Rappleye, Dean at the P&S Medical Center … wanted to have her and her laboratory moved…."

After a week of negotiations, and in response to a plea from the Committee on Administration, McIntosh withdrew his resignation concurrently with the shelving of plans to move the pediatric pathology labs to a location outside Babies Hospital. Douglas Damrosch described the response of the Babies Hospital faculty: "For the staff this was a thrilling demonstration of the Chief's strength" [4]. Richard Day added more succinctly: "Rusty won" [2]. McIntosh's compromise solution was an eventual relocation of the pediatric pathology labs to the Babies Hospital basement.

Several points emerge from this: Dorothy Andersen was essential to McIntosh's vision of Babies Hospital, a vision which included major advances in patient care and research. Andersen had positioned herself both as a successful independent researcher and a popular collaborator for other Babies Hospital faculty and physicians-in-training. Andersen's research – including her ability to attract funding – as well as her expanding role in patient care, with her leadership in the rapidly emerging field of multidisciplinary clinical care required by patients with CF, were explicitly recognized by McIntosh. Her presence in a variety of educational activities at Babies Hospital and beyond was equally important.

In the annual Dean's report of 1950, McIntosh makes reference – somewhat obliquely – to the pediatric pathology problem after it was presumably fixed:

An ominous trend … has become increasingly noticeable over the past several years, namely, the progressive preemption of available laboratory facilities in Babies Hospital by routine diagnostic procedures. Until quite recently, when Presbyterian Hospital generously made available some space for conversion to pediatric laboratories, the only facilities of this sort under direct pediatric supervision were those in the Babies Hospital building. Because of their greater geographical convenience to the staff, these laboratories were for a long time preferred over any in other locations, as in the building of the College of Physicians and Surgeons, which might from time to time be loaned to us for a pediatric project. Now, however, regardless of convenience it is going to be necessary to look beyond the walls of Babies Hospital for areas in which to house selected pediatric research projects which do not depend completely on close proximity to the wards for their successful execution. Limitation of laboratory facilities in the existing situation constitutes a serious handicap in the Department's research program. [5]

This perspective helps frame the argument going forward: the problem of insufficient lab space for research and routine lab work in major medical centers in Manhattan will not be easy to solve. But the critical problem in 1949 was Dorothy Andersen: McIntosh knew how important she was to the mission of Babies Hospital

---

[2] Andersen's CUMC Archive files include very few examples of routine correspondence.

and to the growth of pediatrics generally. He realized that it was likely that some future pediatric research projects would have to be located off-site; but off-site for Dorothy Andersen was not an option that McIntosh would ever consider.

McIntosh's support for Andersen was not conditional on shared perspectives and attitudes: he was at heart conservative in dress and custom, careful to avoid committing himself unless the answer was clear, and more similar in behavior to Holt and an earlier generation than his contemporaries might have realized. Andersen was liberal and less constrained in dress or comportment than her contemporaries, likely to give serious consideration to alternative explanations when she felt that conventional wisdom was unfounded, and more similar in taste and behavior to the younger generation which emerged in her wake in the 1960s. Neither assessment is meant to be pejorative, as there is value in each approach.

Though McIntosh clearly recognized Andersen's value in the major domains associated with academic medicine (clinical care, medical education, and research), he appeared hesitant to sing her praises in public. He coauthored an unpublished history of Babies Hospital several years later in 1953 [1], and in 1963 he presented a brief hospital history at a celebration of the hospital's seventy-fifth anniversary [1]: he did not mention Andersen's landmark CF study in 1938 or the attendant 1939 E. Mead Johnson Award she received,[3] nor any of her "CF firsts." He certainly recognized something exceptional in Andersen that transcended more mundane considerations, but he could not bring himself to declare it as openly as he did for several of her colleagues (like Hattie Alexander), and this suggests that the relationship between Andersen and McIntosh was a bit strained: perhaps they had private disagreements, or just awkward moments (as occurred between McIntosh and Wollstein: "we used to fight over details of laboratory procedure" [1]). This would not be unexpected, given their vastly different temperaments. They were both self-confident with little evidence or need of self-aggrandizement, and both were important figures in the development of pediatrics in the twentieth century; however the relationship between them may not have been close or warm.

By the beginning of the third decade of the McIntosh Era at Babies Hospital, the problem of insufficient laboratory space remained unresolved, though Andersen's own position at Babies Hospital seemed a bit more secure. At least her research and academic heritage – including her "CF firsts" – ensured her a position of honor and respect in the halls of academic medicine.

Maybe.

---

[3] McIntosh was on sabbatical during much of 1940, and the annual report of the Department of Pediatrics to the Dean of Medicine that year was made by Ashley Weech, who noted both Andersen's 1938 study and the 1939 award. McIntosh's earlier reports to the Dean made only vague mention of Andersen's activities (perhaps because her primary allegiance was then still to the Department of Pathology).

References

1. Rustin McIntosh papers. Archives at the Augustus C. Long Health Sciences Library of Columbia University.
2. Straus J, Strauss L. Rusty McIntosh by some of the many who experienced the essence of his presence at Babies Hospital, 1931–1960. Babies Hospital Alumni Association; 1987.
3. Dorothy H. Andersen papers. Archives at the Augustus C. Long Health Sciences Library of Columbia University.
4. Damrosch DS. A tribute to Rustin McIntosh, M.D., C.-P.M. Center, Editor. 1986.
5. Report of the Dean of the School of Medicine. In: Columbia University bulletin of information. New York: Columbia University; 1931–58.

CF Sweat and the Matilda Effect

13

An August heat wave in New York City is a common event, and the absence of air conditioning until at least the 1950s suggests that any associated discomfort in the first half of the twentieth century was much greater during such events compared to currently. The urban heat island effect – in which elevated temperatures in a large urban area may be greater than surrounding rural areas – contributed to an increase in morbidity and mortality associated with these summertime heat waves. In August 1948, a heat wave in New York City was associated with dehydration and heat prostration in ten infants admitted to Babies Hospital: five of these infants had CF, and ongoing surveillance revealed two additional cases with CF and heat prostration during the following two summers.

Walter Kessler, then a senior resident at Babies Hospital, and Dorothy Andersen reported this cohort of children [1]: all were febrile, and those with CF had been vomiting and/or sweating profusely. Hypochloremia[1] was noted in the only two patients who underwent electrolyte testing of their blood; both had CF, and the critical implications related to this finding took years to appreciate.[2] Constraints in available technology limited the blood testing performed on this small series of patients, but Andersen eventually realized that these CF patients were suffering from salt deficiency. Kessler and Andersen suggested that CF patients "are especially susceptible to heat prostration," that hypochloremia was "partly the result of vomiting and partly due to loss of chlorides by sweating," and that CF patients should either avoid high temperatures or "be supplied with large amounts of fluids and additional salt" [1].

---

[1] A low level of chloride in the blood. Hyponatremia (a low level of sodium in the blood) was also noted in one of these patients.

[2] Hypochloremia is associated with metabolic alkalosis in CF, and metabolic alkalosis may lead to worsening respiratory acidosis, a problem which is exacerbated in the presence of severe lung disease as often occurs in CF.

© The Author(s), under exclusive license to Springer Nature Switzerland AG 2022   105
J. S. Baird, *Dorothy Hansine Andersen*,
https://doi.org/10.1007/978-3-030-87484-1_13

Andersen was directly responsible for many of the observations and most of the conclusions in this study focused mainly on heat prostration in CF,[3] including:

> It is of interest to note that some 10 years ago, prior to the advent of antibiotics other than the sulfonamides, several children with cystic fibrosis of the pancreas were taken to areas where warm weather was more constant in order to minimize exposure to respiratory infections. Several of these children died soon after this move, and as a group they did far worse than those who remained in a cooler climate. [1]

Many of the parents of Andersen's patients continued to correspond with her even after they moved away, and Andersen somehow connected the dots in order to guess that warm weather might negatively impact her patients with CF. As a result, one hypothesis the authors suggested was "that the sweat glands, as well as the glands of the pancreas and other organs, are inadequate in function" in CF, entirely consistent with Andersen's earlier contention that "the disease [CF] is a disturbance of many glandular tissues" [2]. If the sweat glands were "inadequate in function", patients with CF might have difficulty coping with a heat wave.

Though Kessler and Andersen were apparently unaware of it, the first model of experimental salt deficiency in humans was developed in the mid-1930s by Robert McCance at King's College Hospital in England, who subjected three volunteers to a salt-free diet coupled with induced sweating using radiant heat [3]. The resultant low levels of sodium and chloride in blood were associated with weakness and cramps, all of which improved rapidly with salt repletion.

The 1951 CF heat prostration study was Andersen's second landmark CF study, though it is much less well-known than her first: it led directly to the three CF sweat studies in 1953, and helped establish a new paradigm for CF. This new paradigm suggested that abnormal loss of chloride via sweat is a hallmark of CF, and this phenomenon was eventually explained in 1983 by Paul Quinton's discovery of the cell membrane channelopathy associated with CF [4]. As a result of the CF heat prostration study, it is clear that Andersen – with her meticulous, orderly approach – made a mental note to investigate her hypothesis about CF sweat further, just like she eventually investigated her vitamin A deficiency hypothesis.

Paul di Sant'Agnese remembered years later: "I took care of these patients as Dr. Andersen was vacationing in England at the time. However, they were reported in the medical literature by Dr. Kessler, at the time the senior resident, and Andersen in 1952 [sic]" [5]. It appears that di Sant'Agnese, an Assistant Pediatrician at Babies Hospital whose major responsibility early in his career was to provide outpatient care for Andersen's CF patients, felt there might have been a problem involving authorship of this study.

Where then was Andersen in the late summer and early fall of 1948? She went to Europe (and returned in time to witness McIntosh's resignation in 1949, as noted in the previous chapter). She described the purpose of her European trip using the third person point of view (which she often used to avoid any hint of self-aggrandizement):

---

[3] Andersen recognized the important contributions of some of the physicians she worked with, like Kessler and di Sant'Agnese, by naming them as first author for a particular study.

> Dorothy Andersen plans to spend the summer in England, if she can get some guarantee of a way to come home again. During the past 2 years a number of English traveling fellows have worked briefly in Dorothy's lab and she is looking forward to visiting them and seeing how they do things over there. [6]

But she also had some bigger plans which she may not have admitted, even to herself:

> It wasn't originally planned as a busman's holiday, but it turned out to be one. When I wrote to various pediatric centers for permission to visit, I was answered by requests to lecture. I ended up by giving papers at the Royal Society of London and the pediatric groups in Manchester, Edinburgh, and Holland. I was rewarded by the best of hospitality, a good time and an interesting one … All in all- an eventful autumn! [6]

She received the Borden award for nutrition research in the late summer of 1948 while she was in Europe [7].

In the decades since Kessler and Andersen reported their findings, di Sant'Agnese's part in the history of CF sweat research has been emphasized. Examples include the following accounts written by physicians with expertise in CF, the first from an online history of clinical care in CF:

> At the time of this report [Kessler and Andersen's study] there was no explanation as to why infants with CF were particularly susceptible to heat prostration and salt depletion – fortunately Paul di Sant'Agnese decided to find out! This was the first report that children with CF were particularly susceptible to heat. It was this original incident that eventually led Paul di Sant'Agnese to search for the reason for salt depletion in many of these CF infants and eventually to his recognising the abnormally high sweat sodium and chloride, and to a lesser extent potassium. This was undoubtedly the first and most important step towards understanding of the causation of CF up to that time. [8]

Another account is from a compendium of reminiscences by some of those who cared for CF patients and/or helped advance our understanding of CF in the twentieth century:

> In 1949, a major heat wave in New York City led to an epidemic of heat prostration in infants …. Dr. Paul di Sant'Agnese at Babies Hospital made the astute observation that the proportion of infants with CF among those with heat prostration was very high, and inferred that there must be some abnormality of the sweat in these infants. He was the first to demonstrate that the salt content of CF sweat was elevated fivefold over normal. [5]

And lastly from a brief review in 2016 of a publication by di Sant'Agnese which appeared 50 years earlier: "She [Andersen] soon enlisted the clinical expertise of Dr. Paul di Sant'Agnese who, following a 1948 summer heat wave, identified sweat chloride abnormality in the condition we now call cystic fibrosis" [9].

The available records suggest some inaccuracies in these three accounts: di Sant'Agnese did not make the observation regarding susceptibility of CF patients to heat prostration; Kessler and Andersen did. Kessler and Andersen were the first to speculate in print that sweating might be responsible for heat prostration in children with CF (and the first reported patients were victims of a heat wave in 1948, not

1949). Andersen enlisted di Sant'Agnese to help provide clinical care for her CF patients and not for any expertise he had with CF; he developed expertise in that disease as a product of her mentorship. And finally, di Sant'Agnese was not the first – or even the principal – author of the first study documenting abnormal sweat electrolytes in CF; that was Robert Darling.

Paolo (later: Paul) Artom di Sant'Agnese was born in Italy in 1914 and graduated from the University of Rome Medical School in 1938. His father, Valerio Artom di Sant'Agnese, was a physician with a practice in obstetrics and gynecology in Rome before World War II:

> Member of a distinguished Italian Jewish family. Artom was gynecologist to the royal family and was raised to the nobility in 1930… Despite the king's intercession with Mussolini and the doctor's previous conversion to Catholicism, Artom was restricted by the anti-Semitic laws from practicing medicine outside the Jewish community. He went into exile in the United States in 1938. [10]

It is likely that royal connections were helpful in allowing the di Sant'Agnese family to emigrate to the United States in 1938.

Royal connections were also involved in Paul di Sant'Agnese's earliest association with Columbia University: a wealthy socialite friend[4] of Columbia University's President Butler asked Butler for help in 1940 with Paul's student status, writing that "H.R.H. … Christopher of Greece … [asked] me to do what I could for him [di Sant'Agnese]" [11]. At the time, di Sant'Agnese was auditing classes at Columbia University's College of Physicians and Surgeons, and it is unclear if Prince Christopher's request had any impact; of course, why the opinions of a European aristocrat regarding a classroom auditor should be communicated to a university president in the United States remains unclear.

Paul di Sant'Agnese later underwent residency training in pediatrics at New York Postgraduate Hospital [12]. During his residency, he published a case report as well as a brief study of vitamin A absorption in infants with eczema, suggesting a possible interest in academic medicine. However, he did not yet have a focus for study, nor did his few publications suggest a particular aptitude for medical research. As an Italian immigrant/refugee, he was unlikely to be drafted for military service in World War II; he was hired by Babies Hospital in 1944 as an assistant pediatrician and as chief of the pediatric clinics at the Vanderbilt Clinic. At the time, Andersen needed someone to help with outpatient CF care, and she may have believed that providing him with mentorship might help him develop some research expertise.

As di Sant'Agnese noted years later: "Dorothy had worked with a pediatrician, Dr. Hodges,[5] who I replaced" [5]. Andersen mentored di Sant'Agnese; she needed a pediatrician who could take care of her CF patients in the clinic, and she gave him research opportunities and a focus for his research. In 1945, his father Valerio Artom di Sant'Agnese died, and in 1946, di Sant'Agnese was himself hospitalized for a

---

[4] Letter from Marion Morgan Kemp.

[5] Hodges collaborated with Andersen on the 1946 study which showed that CF is a genetic disorder behaving in a recessive manner.

severe neurologic disease: acute demyelinating encephalomyelitis. He recovered slowly and was left with some disability. However, he returned to work at Babies Hospital, and he and Andersen completed their 1946 study on antibiotic therapy in CF (reviewed in an earlier chapter). They also completed a general review of CF in 1948 [13]; in both cases, di Sant'Agnese was the first author, a prestigious accomplishment for him.

Also in 1948 di Sant'Agnese completed his doctoral dissertation for a Med. Sc.D. degree from Columbia University. His dissertation was "Combined immunization against Diphtheria, Tetanus, and Pertussis in newborn infants," and this work affirming the newborn's ability to produce antibodies following multiple immunizations led to several publications. Andersen had earned her Med.Sc.D. degree over a decade earlier, and it is likely that her example served as a model for him; he certainly displayed an admirable appetite for work, and Andersen also recognized his apparent aptitude for research.

By the late 1940s, di Sant'Agnese began to investigate glycogen storage diseases and idiopathic celiac disease with Andersen (both topics to be reviewed in later chapters): he was by then included in all of Andersen's most important research efforts, and her mentorship helped define his career.

By 1950 or 1951, it is likely that Andersen and di Sant'Agnese decided on another research project: an investigation of CF sweat. However, during that investigation, something changed in their relationship: the studies in the early 1950s by di Sant'Agnese and Andersen on type II (Pompe) glycogen storage diseases, idiopathic celiac disease, and the first study of CF sweat in 1953 mark the end of Andersen's mentoring relationship with di Sant'Agnese. After the first few months of 1953, di Sant'Agnese would continue his research focus on these same diseases, but his collaborations with Andersen became uncommon.

Any investigation of sweat would certainly benefit from the inclusion of someone with expertise in sweat collection and analysis: Robert Darling was the first Chair of the Department of Rehabilitation Medicine at Columbia University, and he had the expertise. Darling worked with Andre Cournand and Dickinson Richards[6] on a variety of investigations involving cardiorespiratory physiology, as well as on dyshemoglobinemias and their effect on oxygen carriage in blood, but he also studied sweat: one of the technologies he developed was a special room capable of maintaining a constant temperature and humidity [5]. He developed some simple techniques for obtaining sweat and in 1948 reported that sweat from a subject's palm had a chloride concentration that was less than one half the serum concentration in most subjects [14]. Years later di Sant'Agnese commented about sweat chloride that "there were a few reports in the literature about the normal values of these electrolytes [including chloride]" prior to the CF sweat investigations [5]; he neglected to mention that Darling was an influential author of one of these reports. In the CF sweat studies di Sant'Agnese and Andersen were planning, Darling provided the equipment and expertise needed for the investigations. Andersen

---

[6] Cournand and Richards received the Nobel Prize for their exploration of cardiopulmonary physiology, as noted in Chap. 19.

frequently had recourse to experts who assisted her in specific research interests: Alvan Barach in pulmonary medicine, Gerty Cori in biochemistry, and, later in her career, Sidney Blumenthal in pediatric cardiology. It is likely that Robert Darling was another expert she recruited.

This is the context of the investigations into the CF sweat hypothesis which occupied di Sant'Agnese and Andersen for at least 2 years [5] in the early 1950s. It is likely that McCance's experimental model to induce salt deficiency by sweating [3] came to Andersen's attention around this time,[7] and she then realized a more urgent need for this investigation.

The first documented evidence of abnormal sweat electrolytes in CF was published in January 1953 [15]. The last – or senior – author on this study of CF sweat was Andersen; Darling was the first author, while di Sant'Agnese was the second author. At least some of the impetus for this study seemed to originate with Andersen, as suggested by several sentences in the introduction, which referred to the earlier CF heat prostration study:

> Disturbance of the sweating mechanism offers an avenue of explanation which can be explored. Theoretical support is given to this approach by the postulate that the disease [CF] is a disturbance of many glandular tissues. Since the children reported were sweating freely and showed no extreme pyrexia, the mechanism is obviously not that of uncomplicated heat stroke. [15]

The contention that "the disease is a disturbance of many glandular tissues"[8] was an opinion Andersen had offered repeatedly; she had suggested that CF is a "congenital and hereditary defect of the secretion of a number of types of glands" [2]. In this first CF sweat study, nine patients with CF were compared to eight patients without CF (one with no disease, seven with other diseases): sweat sampled from abdominal skin had a "markedly higher concentration of chloride" in the patients with CF.[9] In addition, electrolyte balance data from two adolescents with CF suggested concurrent renal conservation of salt. The authors concluded that "the cause of the excessive salt loss in the sweat probably lies in the sweat glands themselves, a new site for possible abnormality in this disease" [15].

Di Sant'Agnese years later suggested that he had "decided as a 'shot in the dark,' to see if … there was something wrong with the sweat electrolyte concentration [5]" in CF. A recent account seemed to validate di Sant'Agnese's role:

> He [di Sant'Agnese] discovered that other scientists had calculated these values in healthy subjects by placing volunteers in a heated room to induce sweating. He decided to replicate these experiments at Columbia Presbyterian Hospital to see whether children with cystic fibrosis sweated excessively, or if their sweat was chemically different from others. [16]

---

[7] Perhaps from Winifred Young, who trained under McCance around the time he investigated salt deficiency; in the mid-1940s Young also trained in the United States under Andersen and became a close friend.

[8] Though unstated, Andersen's contention focused on exocrine (and not endocrine) glands.

[9] In patients without CF, the sweat chloride was indeed less than one half of the serum value, as Darling's earlier study suggested, while in patients with CF, it was closer to the serum value.

However, this misrepresents the context of this study: Darling had been the one to place volunteers in a heated room at CUMC several years earlier, and Andersen likely recruited him to help investigate her hypothesis about CF sweat. Rather than a "shot in the dark" by di Sant'Agnese, this study was a systematic investigation of Andersen's hypothesis of a defect in CF sweat gland function, and it was completely dependent on Darling's expertise in sweat collection and analysis. The results offered a plausible mechanism for CF patients to develop heat prostration from salt depletion, and the contributions of both Andersen and Darling to this study were uniquely valuable and helped point to a new paradigm for CF pathophysiology. This study was anything but a "shot in the dark."

The next two CF sweat studies were published in November and December of 1953; Di Sant'Agnese was the first author, Andersen was not included, though both studies did include Darling as the second author. Both studies also cited Kessler and Andersen's 1951 CF heat prostration study as well as the first CF sweat study from January 1953. The November 1953 study [17] included forty-three patients with CF vs fifty patients without CF, while the December 1953 study [18] included fifty patients with CF vs fifty patients without CF vs nine patients with non-CF pancreatic disease. Both these studies confirmed an increased sweat chloride concentration associated with CF. All three of the CF sweat studies from 1953 included electrolyte balance data on two adolescents with CF, in which renal conservation of salt during a period of low sodium intake was noted.

Did Andersen contribute to the November and December 1953 studies? And if she did, why wasn't she included as an author? There is no direct evidence, but there are hints. Several of the patients reported in the first study (January 1953) were also reported in the later studies (November and December 1953), and all of the CF patients were from Andersen's CF clinic. Andersen's role as a senior researcher or mentor to di Sant'Agnese over several years seems pretty clear: she included him in nearly all of her research efforts at the time, and this explains, in part, her recognition as the last, or senior author, of the first CF sweat study in January 1953. The role of Andersen's grant funding in support of the three CF sweat studies of 1953 was a bit hazy: all three studies acknowledged support from a United Fruit Company grant to investigate celiac syndrome awarded to Andersen and di Sant'Agnese largely on the basis of Andersen's work before di Sant'Agnese was hired.

Authorship on medical research is a valuable commodity: it may be used to help determine tenure and may be useful to gauge the success of competing researchers and institutions. Authorship also includes an implication of responsibility and accountability, in several directions: certainly toward the study subjects and the data, but also toward the other authors, the institution and/or any sponsor of the study, as well as the journal in which it is published and that journal's audience. There are some rules regarding authorship: formal rules suggest that clinical participation in the care of a patient being reported is not sufficient for inclusion as an author, while informal rules often attribute to the first author much of the credit for the study, and the last author is often considered to be the senior author. If grant money due a senior researcher has been used to help finance a study under the direction of the senior researcher, the senior researcher is assumed to have supervised and been responsible for study procedure and results in compliance with grant requirements, and identifying the grant without including the senior researcher as an author would be a mistake. It is often the case that the senior author/researcher developed a series of ideas, or hypotheses, which help drive the work, independent of any funding, and that these hypotheses include the one driving the investigation under consideration. The senior author often acts as a mentor to help junior faculty achieve first authorship.

The November 1953 study [17] was "the main paper that di Sant'Agnese quoted as describing the sweat electrolyte abnormality" [8]. That study was also described in a history of CF research as "undoubtedly the most important advance in the understanding of CF up to that time" [8]. However, the first published investigation to clearly document abnormal sweat chloride in CF was, in reality, the January 1953 study [15], and this study was omitted entirely from di Sant'Agnese's recollections about the CF sweat investigations [5]. An argument could easily be made that Andersen's CF heat prostration study of 1951 along with the January 1953 CF sweat study were the most important advances in our understanding of CF up to that time, and that these two studies gave birth to a new paradigm in CF.

Regarding the 1953 CF sweat studies: "It is also said that even di Sant' Agnese's close colleague Dorothy Andersen was at first reluctant to accept the findings" [8]. This must, of course, be true: Andersen was always meticulous and demanded rigorous scientific proof before accepting any hypothesis as proven, including her own. It is consistent with her previous work that she would have asked for a complete metabolic profile on several CF patients with abnormal sweat electrolyte results, including renal and adrenal function, and requested that publication be deferred, if needed, until all details were complete. It is likely that she would have requested additional electrolyte balance studies beyond those involving the two adolescents with CF originally reported in the first study and that she would have at least questioned the repeated inclusion of this data from these two adolescents in all three studies. She would certainly have agreed with the study of a larger CF cohort compared to a control group and would likely have suggested other comparisons (perhaps with idiopathic celiac disease). The only surprising result of her meticulous approach to research would be if this somehow reflected negatively upon her.

Unfortunately, in later years questions about Andersen's conduct emerged and some complaints: di Sant'Agnese hinted that he should have been included as an author in the 1951 study by Kessler and Andersen ("I took care of these patients … [5]"), though providing clinical care to patients is not recognized as sufficient criteria for authorship. Philip Farrell, who had worked with di Sant'Agnese for 5 years at the NIH, had "heard him on many occasions describe his experiences of working with Dorothy Andersen" [12]. Farrell then noted that "Andersen lacked the ability to take care of the children that were referred to her," because she "was a pediatric pathologist and not a clinician" [12]. Farrell also noted that "Paul [di Sant'Agnese] had some reluctance to do duodenal drainage studies, because the results … were frightening [12]"[10] and that both Farrell and Lewis Barness felt that Andersen was

---

[10] If true, this would have been an odd perspective for a CF clinical researcher: di Sant'Agnese would have had nothing to study if there were no patients diagnosed with the disease.

difficult and arrogant: "Dorothy Andersen said that she was the only person in the world who really knew about cystic fibrosis back in the late 1930s and even in the 1940s. She was the self-proclaimed expert, and paediatricians of that era, such as Lew Barness, told me that Dorothy travelled around the east coast saying that she really was the only person who knew about cystic fibrosis" [12]. Some years after Andersen's death, di Sant'Agnese even seemed puzzled by Andersen's renown: "how Dr. Andersen, a pathologist, had patients referred to her? I really do not know" [5].

This was extraordinarily disingenuous on his part, as he knew quite well how patients were referred to Andersen: she was designated an Assistant Attending Pediatrician at Babies Hospital by the Department of Pediatrics around the same time di Sant'Agnese was hired, and as an attending pediatrician she had occasional clinical responsibilities on the wards at Babies Hospital. She also evaluated patients referred to her for possible CF before asking di Sant'Agnese – or other pediatricians – to help provide outpatient care. It is likely that Andersen, a meticulous researcher who was not in the habit of leaving her own hypotheses uninvestigated, had a greater role in the CF sweat studies in 1953 than is currently recognized; if so, her role was minimized by di Sant'Agnese.

In 1960, di Sant'Agnese left Babies Hospital and joined the staff of the National Institute of Arthritis, Metabolic and Digestive Diseases at the NIH as the Chief of the Pediatric Metabolism Branch and remained there until retiring. At the NIH he was confronted by another researcher, who said to him about a project they were both working on: "You want me to do the work so that you can write it up" [5]. The Matilda effect[11] is a form of gender bias, in which important scientific discoveries or innovations made by a woman are attributed to a man; undervaluing Andersen's contribution to the 1953 CF sweat studies appears to be an example of the Matilda effect.[12]

The complaints registered by Farrell and Barness are concerning as a manifestation of more overt gender bias: what would they have said if the author of the 1938 CF study was a man? What would they have said if that same man was the first to make a diagnosis of CF in a living patient, the first to report on diet and pancreatic enzyme replacement therapy in CF, and the first to report on the utility of antibiotic therapy in CF? In this context, Andersen *was* the most knowledgeable clinician "about cystic fibrosis back in the late 1930s and even in the 1940s."

Andersen's attitude toward her colleagues and critics was always gracious, and the loyalty she maintained toward her coauthors and colleagues was exemplified by the introduction she wrote for a reprinting of di Sant'Agnese's November 1953 study:

---

[11] Named after Matilda Gage, a famous women's suffragist, by Margaret Rossiter, who first described this phenomenon in 1993.

[12] Author's note: I am unfortunately convinced that Andersen would not agree with this assessment. Her personality and demeanor made her unlikely to engage in confrontation or to blame others if there was any way to avoid or ignore it. I am, however, equally convinced that Andersen's generous nature and lack of interest in confrontations should not contribute to efforts to demean her role in these investigations, and that she was indeed a victim of the Matilda effect.

The most important of the many contributions which he has made to cystic fibrosis was the discovery of the high electrolyte content of the sweat; this has provided our most reliable means of diagnosis and of genetic study of the disease. With enviable exuberance and energy he has explored many other fields productively, notably celiac disease and the glycogen diseases. [19]

Andersen remained supportive of di Sant'Agnese during the remainder of her life. If there was any conflict between them at the time of the CF sweat studies, it is easy to envision her stepping aside graciously, all the while offering approval and support.

She was uninterested in reminding others of her role in the history of CF, though her contributions to the field were by then unrivalled. Her landmark CF studies, including the first accurate disease description in 1938 followed by the heat prostration study in 1951 and the first sweat study in 1953, attest to her skills and intellect and to her meticulous nature. Adding in her "CF firsts" affirms the critical role she had in CF research and care.

Modesty characterized Andersen's approach to her own work, even though the evidence strongly suggests that she knew more about CF in the 1950s than anyone else.

References

1. Kessler WR, Andersen DH. Heat prostration in fibrocystic disease of the pancreas and other conditions. Pediatrics. 1951;8(5):648–56.
2. Andersen DH, Hodges RG. Celiac syndrome; genetics of cystic fibrosis of the pancreas, with a consideration of etiology. Am J Dis Child. 1946;72:62–80.
3. McCance RA. Experimental sodium chloride deficiency in man. Proc R Soc Lond B Biol Sci. 1936;119(814):245–68.
4. Quinton PM. Chloride impermeability in cystic fibrosis. Nature. 1983;301(5899):421–2.
5. Doershuk CF. Cystic fibrosis in the 20th century: people, events, and progress. Cleveland: AM Publishing Ltd; 2001.
6. Dorothy H. Andersen papers. Archives at the Augustus C. Long Health Sciences Library of Columbia University.
7. Sicherman B, Green CH. Notable American women: the modern period: a biographical dictionary. Cambridge, MA: The Belknap Press of Harvard University Press; 1980.
8. Littlewood J. A history of cystic fibrosis. 2002. Available from: www.cysticfibrosismedicine.com.
9. Leung DH, Grand RJ. 50 years ago in the journal of pediatrics: macroscopic cysts of the pancreas in a case of cystic fibrosis. J Pediatr. 2016;176:133.
10. Sarfatti M. My fault: Mussolini as I knew him. New York: Enigma Books; 2014.
11. Babies Hospital historical archives. Archives at the Augustus C. Long Health Sciences Library of Columbia University.
12. Cystic fibrosis witness seminar by the Wellcome Trust for the History of Medicine. London: The Trustee of the Wellcome Trust, UCL; 2002.
13. Di Sant'Agnese PA, Andersen DH. Cystic fibrosis of the pancreas. Prog Pediat Study. 1948;1:160–76.
14. Darling RC. Some factors regulating the composition and formation of human sweat. Arch Phys Med Rehabil. 1948;29(3):150–5.
15. Darling RC, et al. Electrolyte abnormalities of the sweat in fibrocystic disease of the pancreas. Am J Med Sci. 1953;225(1):67–70.

16. Trivedi BP. Breath from salt: a deadly genetic disease, a new era in science, and the patients and families who changed medicine forever. BenBella Books, Incorporated; 2020.
17. Di Sant'Agnese PA, et al. Abnormal electrolyte composition of sweat in cystic fibrosis of the pancreas; clinical significance and relationship to the disease. Pediatrics. 1953;12(5):549–63.
18. Di Sant'Agnese PA, et al. Sweat electrolyte disturbances associated with childhood pancreatic disease. Am J Med. 1953;15(6):777–84.
19. McIntosh R. The McIntosh era at Babies Hospital, 1931–1960: a commemorative volume to honor Rustin McIntosh. Babies Hospital; 1960.

Glycogen Storage Diseases

14

Dorothy Andersen was able to multitask in ways most of the rest of us can only envy. A chapter focused on a particular disease or closely related group of diseases investigated by Andersen might imply that she pursued a series of related investigations sequentially over time, gradually adding to the medical knowledge related to this particular disease or group of diseases, later moving on to investigate something else. In reality, she pursued most of her various research interests nearly simultaneously, so that completely unrelated investigations continued, while she evaluated results and implications of earlier studies (all while she continued her routine work in pathology). For example, in the 1940s while she was working on the studies I have chosen to call her "CF firsts," she was also working on her first study of glycogen storage diseases (below) and her first study of idiopathic celiac disease (next chapter). Such an approach is akin to a juggler attempting to keep several different-sized balls in the air: it requires enormous concentration and skill. She was not always successful in this; her review of pediatric tumors encountered at Babies Hospital from 1935 to 1950 provided a detailed survey of only limited interest [1], and she realized that further work on that topic – like her work on female reproduction in the 1930s – would not lead to major advances. But an autopsy in 1940 helped convince her that glycogen storage diseases would be an interesting topic to investigate further.

The history of glycogen storage diseases must, however, begin with Gerty Radnitz and Carl Cori, who met while they were medical students in Prague. They graduated and married in 1920, emigrated to the United States in 1922, and eventually established themselves at Washington University in St. Louis as an eminently successful research team in biochemistry (though Gerty Cori's career, like Dorothy Andersen's, was also complicated by gender bias and discrimination[1]). The Coris'

---

[1] Though partners at work and co-recipients of the Nobel Prize, Gerty Cori was always paid less than her husband Carl, who also outranked her in the academic hierarchy. Incidentally, Gerty was also a prodigious smoker, like Andersen, and it is likely that the disease responsible for Cori's death in 1958 – myelofibrosis – was in part linked to smoking.

J. S. Baird, *Dorothy Hansine Andersen*,
https://doi.org/10.1007/978-3-030-87484-1_14

discovery in 1939 of the steps involved in muscle breakdown of glycogen (a poly-
mer of glucose residues) to produce energy and lactate and the subsequent reconsti-
tution of glycogen from lactate by the liver (the Cori cycle) led to their shared Nobel
Prize in Physiology or Medicine (1947).

Following that award, Gerty's "greatest interest in her remaining years was the
nature of the enzymatic defects in the glycogen storage diseases" [2]. The specific
enzyme defects leading to abnormal glycogen storage were unknown in the 1940s,
and patients with this problem were then diagnosed with a non-specific eponym:
von Gierke's disease. Over several decades, it became clear that there were probably
several different diseases associated with the syndrome of abnormal glycogen storage, and Cori as well as Andersen and her colleagues all made contributions to this
field. Though these diseases are rare, clarifying the different molecular mechanisms
responsible for these diseases provided an early example of the emerging importance of biochemistry in medicine.

One of Andersen's colleagues was Howard Mason, who trained as an intern
under Luther Emmett Holt, Sr. and worked at Babies Hospital in the 1920s prior to
its move from the east side to the upper west side of Manhattan in 1929 (he was the
one who offered the assessment about how the faculty adjusted to its new surround-
ings "like strange cats"). He was a well-respected academic physician and familiar
with many of the leaders in pediatrics during the first half of the twentieth century.
Mason became interested in pediatric liver disorders, and in late 1939, he helped
care for an infant who died at 3 months of age with hepatomegaly and clinical evidence of von Gierke's disease. Andersen's autopsy of this patient identified glycogen infiltration in the liver and kidneys, and a collaboration on glycogen storage
diseases between Andersen and Mason then continued intermittently for more than
a decade.

They published a detailed case report of this infant in 1941 and used the opportunity to include extensive speculation on the nature of glycogen storage diseases:

> In an effort to identify more exactly the enzyme reaction which was at fault in this case, we
> studied the outline of the steps involved in the transformation of dextrose to glycogen and
> glycogen to dextrose in the liver as recently presented by Cori and his associates. [3]

Though unable to determine a specific enzyme defect in their patient (who likely
had glycogen storage disease type I), Mason and Andersen were convinced that one
of the Cori cycle enzymes was responsible. They reviewed previous reports of von
Gierke's disease, suggesting that it was better to classify it as a syndrome with several clinical types, including:

1. Glycogen storage disease of the liver (true von Gierke's disease), which we
   believe is due to a defect, probably congenital, in one portion of the enzyme
   system of the liver which performs the conversion of glycogen to dextrose and
   dextrose to glycogen...
2. Glycogen storage disease of the heart and muscles. We are inclined to believe
   that in this group the defect is similar but is present at another point in the enzyme
   system [3].

Though their classification was limited by the available biochemical information, their extensive and detailed report revealed excellent clinical skills coupled with an up-to-date knowledge of biochemistry and physiology. In addition, Andersen's foreign language expertise continued to be useful in her medical research, as much of the relevant medical literature regarding glycogen storage diseases was in German, with occasional reports in French or Italian.

In 1950, Mason and Andersen collaborated with Paul di Sant'Agnese and William Bauman on a report of their second type of glycogen storage disease, in which excessive glycogen is found in the heart and muscles. They described the clinical course of two siblings who died with this disorder [4] and reviewed the available medical literature for similar cases [5]. These infants were ultimately accepted as having had glycogen storage disease type II (Pompe disease), though knowledge of the enzyme defect responsible for this disease was not possible for more than a decade following their report.

The first identification of a specific enzyme defect associated with glycogen storage diseases occurred in 1952, and one of Andersen's younger colleagues at Babies Hospital was involved, though she did not receive much credit: Ruth Harris.

Harris had been an undergraduate at Barnard and then earned her M.D. at Columbia in 1943; she finished her pediatric residency training at Babies Hospital in 1946. One of her first studies after joining the Babies Hospital faculty was a report of an extensive treatment plan developed for the care of two children with tetanus in 1948. This treatment included many of the routine therapies currently offered in an ICU long before an ICU would be available at Babies Hospital: sedation, neuromuscular blockade, tracheotomy, as well as a primitive form of mechanical ventilation using a finger [6] (Fig. 14.1).

Both patients survived. Harris had proven herself a clever and dedicated clinician, and this study must have appealed to Andersen, both for its demonstration of steadfast devotion to patient care and for its ingenuity. Subsequently Andersen began an unofficial collaboration with Harris: she provided liver specimens from autopsies or biopsies so that Harris could begin to investigate the amount of specific Cori cycle enzymes present in the tissue.

In 1952, Harris presented evidence of a deficiency of glucose-6-phosphatase in two patients with von Gierke's disease compared to control patients [7]. However, her conclusion was challenged on technical grounds,[2] and a more convincing report of the same deficiency in two patients with von Gierke's disease by Gerty Cori was offered in one of the Harvey lectures[3] that same year [8].

In 1954, Harris coauthored an expanded study of glucose-6-phosphatase levels in children with and without glycogen storage disease [9]; she included data from her preliminary study in 1952, as well as additional data to satisfy critics. She

---

[2] Interestingly, much of the critique was given by Luther Emmett Holt, Jr. (the son of Babies Hospital's first medical director), who also collaborated with Rustin McIntosh on revisions of L.E. Holt, Sr.'s textbook.

[3] An annual series of lectures by leading biomedical researchers offered annually by the Harvey Society in New York City.

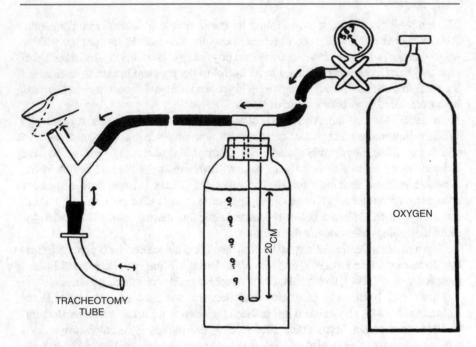

Fig. 14.1 Apparatus for using oxygen under positive pressure via a tracheotomy tube [6]. (Courtesy of Pediatrics)

concluded that glucose-6-phosphatase "activity in two cases of glycogen storage disease of the liver was almost absent, while the liver enzyme activity in one case of glycogen storage disease of the heart was abnormally high" [9]. "Glycogen storage disease of the liver" was soon renamed: glycogen storage disease type I, or "true" von Gierke's disease (as suggested years earlier by Mason and Andersen).

In 1955 Mason and Andersen reported on the clinical course of a debilitated child with type I glycogen storage disease who died at 10 years of age [10]; this was one of the two patients that Harris had reported in 1952 (and Gerty Cori had also included this patient in her Harvey lecture). As might be expected from knowledge of what a defect in the Cori cycle would lead to: "Blood lactate was consistently elevated, the degree of elevation bearing an inverse relationship to blood sugar levels" [10]. As a result, alternative tissue sources were used to provide energy in this patient who was unable to significantly increase her blood glucose in response to muscle activity: "The concentration of total serum lipids was always high... probably reflecting the mobilization of body fat during these periods [of hypoglycemia]" [10]. Mason and Andersen helped to define the natural history of this new disease, associated in their patient with episodes of hypoglycemia and resultant growth failure as well as cognitive dysfunction.

Another Columbia University connection to the history of glycogen storage diseases was Joseph Larner, who graduated from Columbia University's College of Physicians and Surgeons in 1945 and later studied in the Cori Laboratory at Washington University. He described the results of an experiment on a tissue sample from a patient with von Gierke's disease:

I first considered and then proposed to Gerty the possibility that the disease—then considered to be a single ailment termed Von Gierke's disease—might be due to a lack of the debranching enzyme, amylo-1,6- glucosidase. But Gerty felt that the missing enzyme was glucose 6-phosphatase. Behind us in the laboratory stood a chemical cabinet that contained, among other things, a set of glycogen samples Gerty had isolated from tissues sent to her by numerous clinical investigators interested in this disease. I reasoned that, if I were correct, the glycogen itself would have an abnormal structure, with shortened outer chains, but with branch points intact. If Gerty were correct, the glycogen structure would be normal. We made a wager on the outcome—a common event in the laboratory. With her permission I proceeded to take one of the glycogen samples from the cabinet, dissolve a small aliquot in water, and stain it with a few drops of iodine solution in a test tube. To both Gerty's and my amazement, the sample stained bluish-purple with iodine—more like a starch than a glycogen! This sample had been sent by Dorothy Anderson, my former pediatrics teacher from Columbia University College of Physicians and Surgeons. [2]

The unusual nature of Andersen's sample was due to the patient's specific enzyme defect, which was a deficiency in the branching enzyme which helps make normal human glycogen.

By the mid-1950s, Mason was in his late 70s, and his activities became progressively more limited.[4] As a result, in 1956 Andersen was the sole author of a case report on the clinical course of this patient with a new type of glycogen storage disease: a 1-year-old male who died with a febrile illness and cirrhosis associated with an unusual type of glycogen deposited in the liver and the reticuloendothelial system. Following Larner's dramatic demonstration that this patient's glycogen behaved more like starch than glycogen, as well as the Cori's chemical analysis of this patient's glycogen [11], it became clear that this was the first report of disease secondary to deficient glycogen branching enzyme, or glycogen storage disease type IV (hence the disease eponym: Andersen's disease) [12].

In 1958 just a few months after her death, Gerty Cori's summary of her investigations into glycogen storage diseases provided a preliminary classification of the first four types of glycogen storage disease [13]: direct evidence of the enzyme defects were noted for type I (von Gierke's disease) and type III (Cori disease), while indirect evidence at that time suggested the enzyme defect in type IV (Andersen disease). Though type II (Pompe disease) appeared also to be a separate clinical type, no evidence of an enzyme defect was then available (and indeed identification of the lysosomal enzyme defect responsible for this type did not occur until the next decade). The speculation offered by Mason and Andersen in 1941 about the relationship between glycogen storage diseases and the Cori cycle enzymes was indeed prescient. Additional types and subtypes of glycogen storage disease have been identified in the decades since, all of which are related to enzyme defects in the Cori cycle (or in glycolysis).

In 1962 after di Sant'Agnese's move to the NIH, he and Andersen with Kenneth Metcalf published a report of a child who died with an unknown type of glycogen storage disease involving mainly the muscles [14]: beyond ruling out several of the

---

[4] He spent his entire career at Babies Hospital and at his death was described as "a doctor's doctor."

known types, neither di Sant'Agnese nor Cori's laboratory[5] in St. Louis was able to further characterize the disease. By this time, Andersen's own interest in a deeper exploration of glycogen storage diseases had waned, and di Sant'Agnese's plan to utilize basic science researchers at the NIH to help characterize metabolic defects in glycogen storage diseases apparently came to nought [15].

A review of the studies of glycogen storage diseases by the Coris, Harris, Mason, di Sant'Agnese, and Andersen suggests the mostly collaborative nature of their research efforts. Because these diseases are rare, tissue specimens are therefore of great value. But as a result, some confusion about tissue sources was apparent in many of the early studies, and occasional patients were reported by several different authors in different publications at different times. Andersen's explanation of how she handled the specimens from one such patient helped clarify how different investigators might all contribute results over several years for the same patient:

> Aliquots of liver, liver tumor and kidney were given at once to Dr. Ruth C. Harris for glucose-6-phosphatase determination, and other portions of these tissues were frozen and at a later date sent for analysis to Dr. Gerty Cori. [10]

Indeed, this patient with glycogen storage disease type I (WM) was reported at different times by Harris [7, 9], Mason and Andersen [10], as well as Cori [8]. Using different lab methodologies, Harris and Cori performed enzyme assays which affirmed the enzymatic defect: "Both Dr. Cori and Dr. Harris found a striking diminution in glucose-6-phosphatase" [9]. As this patient was one of the two patients reported in Harris' 1952 study and the same patient was included in Cori's Harvey lecture that year, Harris' 1952 results were actually validated by Cori.

Later in Harris' career, she occasionally revisited the glycogen storage diseases, but only peripherally. Her research interests by then had changed to include the various causes of neonatal and infant cholestasis as well as portal hypertension in children, though she also enjoyed exploring a broad range of other rare and/or poorly understood diseases; in some ways, her approach and interests recall Andersen's and suggest a kindred spirit.

While Andersen and Mason deserve credit for their early attempt to separate and categorize different glycogen storage diseases in 1941, and Andersen deserves additional credit for mentoring di Sant'Agnese for their study of type II (Pompe) disease as well as for her own identification of type IV (Andersen) disease, Gerty Cori remains the individual most responsible for our current understanding of these diseases, including the relevant metabolic pathways. Understanding these diseases in the 1940s and 1950s helped ensure that biochemistry would occupy a critical place in the practice of medicine from then on.

And Andersen contributed to that new paradigm.

---

[5] Following Gerty Cori's death from myelofibrosis, Barbara Illingworth-Brown continued biomedical research into the causes of glycogen storage diseases at Washington University and was able to do a partial analysis of this patient's glycogen.

References

1. Andersen DH. Tumors of infancy and childhood. I. A survey of those seen in the pathology laboratory of the Babies Hospital during the years 1935-1950. Cancer. 1951;4(4):890–906.
2. Larner J. Gerty Theresa Cori: August 8, 1896-October 26, 1957. Biogr Mem Natl Acad Sci. 1992;61:111–35.
3. Mason HH, Andersen DH. Glycogen disease. Am J Dis Child. 1941;61(4):795–825.
4. Di Sant'Agnese PA, et al. Glycogen storage disease of the heart. I. Report of 2 cases in siblings with chemical and pathologic studies. Pediatrics. 1950;6(3):402–24.
5. Di Sant'Agnese PA, Andersen DH, Mason HH. Glycogen storage disease of the heart. II. Critical review of the literature. Pediatrics. 1950;6(4):607–24.
6. Harris RC, McDermott TR, Montreuil FL. The treatment of tetanus. Pediatrics. 1948;2(2):175–85.
7. Harris RC. Preliminary studies of liver glucose-6-phosphatase in von Gierke's disease. Am J Dis Child. 1952;84(5):627–8.
8. Cori GT. Glycogen structure and enzyme deficiencies in glycogen storage disease. Harvey Lect. 1952;48:145–71.
9. Harris RC, Olmo C. Liver and kidney glucose-6-phosphatase activity in children with normal and diseased organs. J Clin Invest. 1954;33(9):1204–9.
10. Mason HH, Andersen DH. Glycogen disease of the liver (von Gierke's disease) with hepatomata; case report with metabolic studies. Pediatrics. 1955;16(6):785–800.
11. Cori GT, Cori CF. Glucose-6-phosphatase of the liver in glycogen storage disease. J Biol Chem. 1952;199(2):661–7.
12. Andersen DH. Familial cirrhosis of the liver with storage of abnormal glycogen. Lab Investig. 1956;5(1):11–20.
13. Cori GT. Biochemical aspects of glycogen deposition disease. Bibl Paediatr. 1958;66:344–58.
14. Di Sant'Agnese PA, Andersen DH, Metcalf KM. Glycogen storage disease of the muscles. Report of a case with unusual features. J Pediatr. 1962;61:438–42.
15. Doershuk CF. Cystic fibrosis in the 20th century: people, events, and progress. Cleveland: AM Publishing Ltd; 2001.

Idiopathic Celiac Disease

15

It is possible to trace some of Dorothy Andersen's early work on CF back to Luther Emmett Holt, Sr. as a result of his interest in the celiac syndrome: this syndrome then included patients with CF as well as others with true celiac disease, which is an enteropathy[1] we now know to be associated with gluten exposure in genetically susceptible individuals. The history of celiac syndrome is interwoven with the history of Babies Hospital: it was, after all, an autopsy at Babies Hospital of a child with celiac syndrome and an abnormal pancreas that led Andersen in 1935 to recognize CF as a new disease distinct from celiac disease. But decades earlier, Holt had some expertise with celiac syndrome, as is clear from this anecdote provided by Rustin McIntosh:

> About 1900 my sister, then a young girl, had digestive trouble which baffled the local practitioners in Omaha. (In retrospect, I surmise that she had a mild grade of coeliac disease.) She was brought, in desperation, all the way to New York to see Dr. Holt. Therapy took the form of a regulated way of life, including a strict diet which avoided sugar and most forms of starch. The symptomatic response was so gratifying as to demonstrate clearly that Dr. Holt knew what he was dealing with. After some weeks and months of encouraging improvement my sister was so greatly changed from her former state that my mother, looking ahead, was emboldened to write to Dr. Holt to ask his sanction for a special Christmas celebration, a departure from the strict diet to the extent of permission for one (:1) piece of candy. I'm sure that my mother looked on this one anticipated treat as a symbol of Peace on Earth, Good Will Toward Men.
>
> The reply, written in Dr. Holt's hand, has alas not been preserved, but was said to have run as follows:
>
> My dear Mrs. McIntosh: Why you should wish to make your daughter ill on Christmas rather than on any other day I fail to understand.
>
> Yours faithfully, L. Emmett Holt. [1]

---

[1] A disease of the intestines

© The Author(s), under exclusive license to Springer Nature Switzerland AG 2022
J. S. Baird, *Dorothy Hansine Andersen*,
https://doi.org/10.1007/978-3-030-87484-1_15

While serving as the Chair of Pediatrics at Columbia University's College of Physicians and Surgeons, Holt apparently was also responsible for encouraging Christian Herter, John Howland, and Sidney Haas to investigate celiac syndrome [2]:

- In 1908, Herter suggested that an abnormal intestinal bacterial flora and consumption of carbohydrates might be responsible. He preferred the name "intestinal infantilism" to describe this syndrome [3] – a reflection of the abnormal intestinal bacterial flora.
- In 1921, Howland (later the Chair of Pediatrics at Johns Hopkins) suggested that a restriction of dietary carbohydrates was therapeutic.
- In 1924, Haas reported that a diet restricted in carbohydrates – except for banana – was beneficial in eight patients with celiac syndrome. The banana diet then became an important therapeutic option for the disease.

The conclusion of all three researchers – that carbohydrates, with the possible exception of bananas, might be associated with the symptoms of celiac syndrome – was consistent with Holt's advice to McIntosh's mother, though far from a determination of the actual cause of any of the diseases responsible for the syndrome.

Hattie Alexander began her career at Babies Hospital with an investigation into the celiac syndrome in the early 1930s: she reviewed laboratory results and clinical findings from a group of these patients at Beth Israel Hospital in New York City [4]. Though this investigation did not result in a publication, Rustin McIntosh believed Alexander's work was beneficial:

> One of her [Alexander's] first investigative efforts was to take a look at the intestinal flora of celiac patients, more or less repeating – but with more sophisticated bacteriological methods – a study made by Christian A. Herter of the Rockefeller Institute earlier in the century. Nothing new came of her efforts. But all the while the routine diagnostic work was being improved. [5]

While Andersen's interest in celiac syndrome was originally linked to her recognition of CF as a separate disease, she maintained an interest in celiac syndrome throughout her career. She was certainly aware of the earlier work by Herter, Howland, and Haas, and she became convinced of the benefits of Haas' banana diet in the treatment of celiac syndrome – whether or not it was associated with CF – early in her career. It was indeed the potential benefit of dietary bananas that helped push the United Fruit Company to support several of Andersen's research projects, most of which were focused on CF. In her landmark 1938 CF study, she recommended that patients with CF be treated with a "diet for celiac disease" [6], and by 1945 she clarified that to mean a diet high in calories but low in fat and suggested that "carbohydrate is given to marasmic infants in the form of dextrose and bananas or banana powder" [7].

When a causal mechanism has been identified in patients with a particular syndrome, those patients with this new disease are then considered separately from others with the syndrome: Andersen's identification of CF as a separate disease in 1938 meant that CF patients might have many of the signs and symptoms of other patients with celiac syndrome, but they actually had CF, and for scientific and medical purposes should be considered separately. Once CF patients are excluded from the celiac syndrome, the remaining patients might have another identifiable disease – which could be called "idiopathic celiac disease" for want of a better name: this was Andersen's hypothesis, and she pursued it in 1947 [8] and again in 1953 [9] with Paul di Sant'Agnese. She defined the signs and symptoms of idiopathic celiac disease in young children as chronic or recurrent diarrhea without an underlying cause or identifiable disease but with abdominal distention, failure to thrive, and improvement associated with dietary therapy [8].

Andersen's 1947 study included eighty-five young children: she noted episodic steatorrhea associated with symptomatic worsening (hence the revised clinical definition she used in the next study). She also noted persistent starch intolerance in a subset of patients with decreased pancreatic secretion of amylase and undigested fecal starch, though she did not believe that decreased amylase secretion was responsible for the disease. In order to avoid exacerbations, she suggested that "Cereal starches, bread, and potatoes are withheld for a year or more after recovery from the severe symptoms" [8]. Though it was not possible to identify a cause for this disease, Andersen suspected that something in this group of starchy foods was likely associated with disease exacerbations. Starch consists mainly of carbohydrates, and maintaining an adequate intake of carbohydrates while avoiding these starchy foods was possible, Andersen believed, using a diet rich in bananas and fruit juices.

Her 1953 study with di Sant'Agnese included fifty-eight young children: they again found some evidence of decreased pancreatic secretion of amylase, but nothing to contradict the observations and recommendations she made in her 1947 study. They were still unable to find a causal mechanism or even any clues which might suggest future investigations. The work the authors put into the numerous lab investigations performed on these patients (measurement of pancreatic enzymes in duodenal secretions, glucose tolerance testing, vitamin and protein levels in the blood, and stool analysis for fat) was daunting, and the mostly normal results must have been frustrating.

However, the etiology of celiac disease began to emerge in the early 1950s from an unlikely source: Willem Dicke, a Dutch pediatrician, had become convinced of the central role of wheat, mainly as a result of careful consideration of the dietary responses of individual patients. Like Andersen's CF study in 1938, a better understanding of celiac disease apparently also started with a single patient [10]. After careful but uncontrolled clinical trials in his celiac disease patients, he was able to show the benefits of a wheat-free diet in 1941 (published in a Dutch medical journal), and he then began systematic investigations of various wheat fractions to attempt to isolate the offending agent.

An interesting story emerged following World War II which suggested a possible clue in the celiac disease puzzle to those who were not reading Dutch medical journals: Andersen noted [8] that a decrease in nutritional variety (i.e., fewer fruits and vegetables) was a common problem in many European cities (like Copenhagen) early during the war, along with an increased incidence of celiac disease flares. By the winter of 1944–1945, with even less nutritional support and variety available in much of Europe (including Copenhagen), fewer celiac disease flares were noted – including by Dicke, at least until bread was airdropped into Holland. In retrospect, a greater reliance on bread to supply nutritional needs early in the war was followed by a scarcity of bread later in the war; wheat was thus suspected of a central role in celiac disease flares. However, as Dicke had already concluded that wheat contained a toxic component associated with celiac disease, this wartime observation was not the first bit of evidence to suggest the wheat hypothesis[10]; it does, however, make a good story.

Dicke's thesis in 1950 described in more detail the effect of various diets on patients with celiac disease. By 1953, Dicke and coworkers showed that the toxic component of wheat was a protein complex: gluten. Though carbohydrates make up most of the nutritional content of wheat flour, some protein (including gluten) is also present in small amounts. While Andersen had suggested that diets relying on starch were associated with the underlying cause of celiac disease, it was only after Dicke identified the gluten protein present in various grains as the culprit that this association was understood, and celiac disease was no longer described as idiopathic.

Andersen and di Sant'Agnese's 1953 study on idiopathic celiac disease appeared the same year as the three CF sweat studies, a year after Andersen's extensive review of childhood tumors [11], 2 years after Kessler and Andersen's CF heat prostration study [12], and 3 years after di Sant'Agnese and Andersen's study on type II glycogen storage [13, 14]. It is easy to imagine that both Andersen and di Sant'Agnese were a bit overextended at this point; perhaps they were a bit tired of each other, or perhaps there was some conflict which rendered further collaborations less likely. Like McIntosh, di Sant'Agnese was conservative in dress and custom, perhaps even more so than McIntosh: his connections to European aristocracy were an important part of his personal history, while Andersen's liberal nature suggested that she was unlikely to consider such connections important.

In any case, Andersen pursued another hypothesis regarding celiac disease with Paul Boyer in 1956 [15]: they evaluated the pedigrees of 50 young children with celiac disease and concluded there was no statistically significant increase in the incidence of diabetes in patients with celiac disease, though their conclusion was nuanced [15]:

> The possibility of an association between the incidence of celiac disease and the incidence of diabetes ... was not confirmed. Such a relationship seems unlikely, but no definite conclusions could be reached from the evaluation of the figures obtained in this study. [15]

The role of autoimmunity in celiac disease is now better characterized, and the incidence of type I diabetes (and other autoimmune diseases) is increased in patients with celiac disease and their families, suggesting that Boyer and Andersen's nuance was justified.

Long after Haas' 1924 study and Holt's death, Andersen continued to rely on the banana diet to treat patients with CF: in the early 1950s, Doris Tulcin – whose daughter was diagnosed with CF by Andersen (Chap. 11) – noted that:

Dr. Andersen had discovered a banana formula, called Probana. She had been working on a United Fruit Company grant and prescribed eating only bananas, strained meat out of a baby jar, and the formula for 1 year. Pancreatin was added as the pancreatic enzyme replacement for digestion, vitamins, and Gantrisin as the antibiotic. [16]

It was this United Fruit Company grant that was cited in the three CF sweat studies of 1953. Probana was developed as a pediatric formula and eventually trademarked in 1949. It turns out that banana has no gluten, and the carbohydrates in bananas may be more easily digested compared to other fruits; the banana diet recommended by Andersen to Tulcin was less toxic to patients with idiopathic celiac disease. However specific benefits of the banana diet for CF patients are not as easy to identify, and it is not used much currently.

By 1955, Andersen was convinced by Dicke's thesis of the benefits of avoiding wheat in patients with celiac disease [17]. However, Dicke's discovery – like Andersen's meticulous work in CF – though vital, represented only the first step to a better understanding of the disease. The role of genetic and autoimmune factors in celiac disease is complex [18], and it is likely that continued investigation will disclose additional factors which contribute to its incidence, including intestinal bacterial flora, infant breastfeeding practices, and certain gastrointestinal infections [18]. It is even possible that continued research will find unsuspected links between celiac disease and CF, including a role for CFTR defects in both diseases [19].

Though Andersen was unsuccessful at advancing our knowledge of celiac disease, and was wrong about an association between celiac disease and diabetes, she nevertheless developed remarkable expertise in pediatric nutrition: her use of Haas' banana diet did help many of her patients with the celiac syndrome, her work on CF dietary therapy was an early step in therapeutic interventions to prolong life in CF, and her work on the vitamin A deficiency hypothesis in CF – using an animal model – helped show that maternal dietary deficiency could influence the expression of a congenital malformation (congenital diaphragmatic hernia) in an animal model. As already mentioned, she received the Borden Award for nutrition research from the American Academy of Pediatrics in 1948. Her experience affirmed the importance of laboratory investigations for many patients with a nutrition disorder, as she noted at a luncheon in 1958 honoring her work:

It is usually possible to find out through laboratory research just what the trouble is and what nutrition is needed to act intelligently about it. The trial and error method, changing a bottle formula ... used to be the only method of treating indigestion in infants. Now, if the baby does not recover soon after this treatment, we can apply laboratory methods to discover what is wrong. And we can prescribe accordingly. [20]

By 1958, the role of the laboratory in medical care was rapidly expanding: not only would it be the site of active research into basic science mechanisms responsible for human disease, but Andersen believed it could also be used to help guide care for individual patients. Her vision of pediatric care in this context was hopeful and logical: but it was, nevertheless, only a vision. Changing infant formulas for "intolerance" remains a common practice decades after Andersen's death.

References

1. Mason HH, Park EA. Luther Emmet Holt, 1855-1924. J Pediatr. 1956;49(3):342–69.
2. Haas SV. Celiac disease. N Y State J Med. 1963;63:1346–50.
3. Abel EK. The rise and fall of celiac disease in the United States. J Hist Med Allied Sci. 2010;65(1):81–105.
4. Hattie E. Alexander papers. Archives at the Augustus C. Long Health Sciences Library of Columbia University.
5. Rustin McIntosh papers. Archives at the Augustus C. Long Health Sciences Library of Columbia University.
6. Andersen DH. Cystic fibrosis of the pancreas and its relation to celiac disease: a clinical and pathologic study. Am J Dis Chil. 1938;56(2):344–99.
7. Andersen DH. Celiac syndrome: III. Dietary therapy for congenital pancreatic deficiency. Am J Dis Child. 1945;70(2):100–13.
8. Andersen DH. Celiac syndrome; the relationship of celiac disease, starch intolerance, and steatorrhea. J Pediatr. 1947;30(5):564–82.
9. Andersen DH, Di Sant'Agnese PA. Idiopathic celiac disease. I. Mode of onset and diagnosis. Pediatrics. 1953;11(3):207–23.
10. Yan D, Holt PR. Willem Dicke. Brilliant clinical observer and translational investigator. Discoverer of the toxic cause of celiac disease. Clin Transl Sci. 2009;2(6):446–8.
11. Andersen DH. Tumors of infancy and childhood. Bull N Y Acad Med. 1952;28(7):480–1.
12. Kessler WR, Andersen DH. Heat prostration in fibrocystic disease of the pancreas and other conditions. Pediatrics. 1951;8(5):648–56.
13. Di Sant'Agnese PA, et al. Glycogen storage disease of the heart. I. Report of 2 cases in siblings with chemical and pathologic studies. Pediatrics. 1950;6(3):402–24.
14. Di Sant'Agnese PA, Andersen DH, Mason HH. Glycogen storage disease of the heart. II. Critical review of the literature. Pediatrics. 1950;6(4):607–24.
15. Boyer PH, Andersen DH. A genetic study of celiac disease; incidence of celiac disease, gastrointestinal disorders, and diabetes in pedigrees of children with celiac disease. AMA J Dis Child. 1956;91(2):131–7.
16. Doershuk CF. Cystic fibrosis in the 20th century: people, events, and progress. Cleveland: AM Publishing Ltd; 2001.
17. Andersen DH, Mike EM. Diet therapy in the celiac syndrome. J Am Diet Assoc. 1955;31(4):340–6.
18. Lebwohl B, Sanders DS, Green PHR. Coeliac disease. Lancet. 2018;391(10115):70–81.
19. Villella VR, et al. A pathogenic role for cystic fibrosis transmembrane conductance regulator in celiac disease. EMBO J. 2019;38(2):e100101.
20. Dorothy H. Andersen papers. Archives at the Augustus C. Long Health Sciences Library of Columbia University.

Randomized Clinical Trials

16

Dorothy Andersen's research interests broadened in the last decade of her career as she continued to initiate investigations of several different diseases (or closely related groups of diseases) nearly simultaneously. Her statistical expertise was critical to this research; she even shared her statistical expertise with colleagues.[1] However, Andersen was well aware of the limitations of statistical analyses. Her experiences reporting the earliest results of CF treatment (her "CF firsts") suggested to her some of the flaws of retrospective analyses of therapeutic efficacy: it was difficult to compare outcomes without a control group, confounding variables could greatly limit any analysis, and it was difficult to account for bias.

Late in her career, she was involved in a new type of research methodology: randomized clinical trials (RCTs), championed by her colleagues William Silverman and Richard Day. Silverman and Day advocated strongly for this new research methodology: a group of patients with a specific disease or condition are randomly assigned either to a routine (i.e., control) therapy or a new therapy. If the two groups are similar before treatment, then any difference after treatment may indicate which therapy is better, as long as the groups are large enough to account for confounding variables, and research bias is limited (easy to say, not so easy to do).

Both Silverman and Day – Day served in part as Silverman's mentor but also as his partner in these investigations – became convinced of the necessity of RCTs in neonatology and in medicine generally.[2] They advocated so strongly for RCTs that some of the faculty felt they were annoying. Those faculty members who remained unconvinced apparently did have a point, as related years later by Silverman:

> When Dick Day and I were driving everyone crazy with our emphasis on statistics, clinical epidemiology and numbers, Jack Caffey, at one point got so exasperated, he said, "Bill, I

---

[1] Andersen mentored Hilde Bruch in statistics for Bruch's studies on childhood obesity in 1939. She also mentored several physicians in statistics for several of her CF studies.

[2] In the last few decades, disadvantages to RCTs have also been described, including expense, sample size, and ethical considerations, among others. Controversy exists about the relative value of labor-intensive RCTs vs other study types.

© The Author(s), under exclusive license to Springer Nature Switzerland AG 2022
J. S. Baird, *Dorothy Hansine Andersen*,
https://doi.org/10.1007/978-3-030-87484-1_16

wouldn't believe it even if you proved it to me." ... as the years went by I realized he was absolutely right; there are no complete proofs here in medicine. [1]

Andersen's contribution to the emergence of this new research methodology at Babies Hospital requires a caveat: she was only a minor participant in the story, and her role was centered on her expertise as a pathologist and not on any expertise with statistics or research methodology. Nevertheless, she did contribute in spite of limited available time and numerous other projects. Though she knew as well as anyone else that "there are no complete proofs here in medicine," she must have felt that there was more potential benefit than exasperation in this new approach. This episode also offers a small window into the interests and concerns of some of her Babies Hospital colleagues.

Silverman was one of the most influential neonatologists in the second half of the twentieth century, in large part as he championed this new type of academic research: "a neonatologist, [he] became a trialist the hard way; seeing his tiny patients suffer and die because he and his colleagues either didn't know what to do, or thought they knew more than they did, a situation probably no less true today than 50 years ago" [2]. With the emergence of the subspecialty of neonatology, many common practices for newborn infants needed to be tested to see if they actually helped or hurt. And with technologic advances leading to an increase in the survival of some premature infants, a subsubspecialty involving care of the tiniest and most premature infants emerged. These infants often suffer from morbidities which were unknown only a few years earlier, such as blindness or chronic lung disease. When several premature infants who appeared to be developing retinopathy of prematurity (ROP; a condition which may lead to blindness) appeared to get better following treatment with adrenocorticotropic hormone[3] (ACTH), Silverman and Day were confronted with a dilemma: publish their own case series showing the improved outcome associated with ACTH or insist on a more rigorous clinical trial, as the side effects of ACTH were pernicious. "There was, nonetheless, tremendous pressure to publish our experience. Word had leaked out that we had a spectacular cure for ROP- it was being used in Rhode Island, in Boston, and in Chicago. Dorothy Andersen told us that her friend Beryl Corner,[4] a pediatrician in Bristol, England, was using ACTH" [3]. Word "leaked out" in a publication by Silverman and Day, who described their success using ACTH [4].

However, the two authors then had a kind of epiphany (which suggested remorse), as reported years later by Silverman:

> The 2 of us began to criticize everyone's work because they were making observational studies and no experimental studies, making ourselves a nuisance about our preoccupation with medical statistics. And now here we were with an observational study with no concurrent controls! This was particularly worrisome because of the horrendous side-effects of ACTH. What should we do now? We found ourselves hoist on our own petard! [1]

---

[3] A hormone which is released by the pituitary and stimulates the production and release of cortisol from the adrenal glands.

[4] Corner was one of the founders of neonatology in Great Britain.

Early in 1950 Silverman and Day began to consider a more rigorous clinical test: they considered an investigation of ACTH with an RCT. Discussions of the role of ACTH at academic society meetings as well as at Babies Hospital helped push Silverman and Day, and they eventually presented their ideas to Rustin McIntosh:

> At this point we went to see Rusty and poured out the unhappy story. We told him that we could not, in good conscience, publish the results until ACTH was put to a credible test. The model we had in mind was the first-of-its-kind randomized clinical trial designed by Bradford Hill to compare bed rest (the accepted treatment for early tuberculosis) with strep-tomycin (then a newly proposed drug). The report of this pioneering trial had been pub-lished just two years earlier.... Here, we argued, was a cautious, highly efficient, and, above all, a fair plan... Rusty sat there for a while, puffing on the pipe he smoked in those days. Finally he said "You must do it." For me, this was the moment of truth about Babies Hospital. Rusty emphasized the word <u>must</u>, and it spoke volumes about the BH spirit. [3]

Silverman and Day's first RCT in 1952 was one of the first in neonates – or chil-dren – anywhere and was also one of the first RCTs in the United States: a trial of ACTH in the treatment of ROP in two New York City hospitals (Babies Hospital and Lincoln Hospital) [5]. They found that ACTH did not alter the outcome from ROP compared to untreated infants, but was associated with an increased risk of infection and growth inhibition. After this RCT, ACTH was no longer routinely recommended to treat ROP in premature infants.

Then as evidence began to emerge implicating supplemental oxygen in the devel-opment of ROP, Silverman and Day – among many other physicians – argued for another RCT to address this question. Beginning in 1952, an RCT involving 18 hospitals – including Babies Hospital – was initiated to investigate the effect of supplemental oxygen on the development of ROP in premature infants. The results were published in 1955 and confirmed an increased risk of ROP in premature infants associated with an inspired oxygen concentration greater than 50 percent during the first few weeks of life [6]. The use of routine supplemental oxygen therapy in pre-mature infants was subsequently limited, and Dorothy Andersen would certainly have been intrigued by this result. It was, for Silverman, the signal for a new approach to neonatology: "Beginning in 1954, we outlined an ongoing series of clinical trials to try and narrow the area of uncertainty about almost every aspect of neonatal care" [3].

Silverman's next three RCTs were all performed in collaboration with Dorothy Andersen, beginning with a test of a misted detergent (Alevaire; which was assumed to function as a surfactant to help eliminate mucus secretions in airways) in incuba-tors of premature infants to prevent neonatal respiratory distress syndrome. They reported in 1955 that "there was no therapeutic benefit as judged by death rate and autopsy findings that could be credited to Alevaire mist therapy of premature infants in the first three days of life" [7]. So this therapy was abandoned. Their second RCT in 1956 showed no benefit of a water mist vs a high humidity environment in incu-bators of premature infants at Babies Hospital, and so water mist was abandoned [8].

In 1956, Silverman and Andersen reported the results of their third RCT in col-laboration with William Blanc and Douglas Crozier: this was a comparison of regimens for antibiotic prophylaxis in premature infants at Babies Hospital. According to Silverman, "I wanted the medical students and the house officers at Babies to get more experience with randomized trials, so I proposed that they conduct this antibiotic trial. They all refused, 'Too dull.' They said it isn't interesting enough" [1]. It turned out to be quite interesting: the older regimen of penicillin with sulfisoxazole was associated with a higher mortality rate and an increased incidence of kernicterus compared to the newer regimen of tetracycline [9]. The results were so unexpected that they apparently were not believed by one of the investigators:

> Silverman has recounted that, "after completing a draft describing the trial, I asked the neuropathologist who had examined the brain sections blindly to review the manuscript. I indicated that his name and those of the pediatric pathologists should appear on the paper as co-authors. To my astonishment, when he returned the draft, he said that he did not want his name on the report because the findings were too bizarre! He was sure I was being misled by 'mere statistics'..." [10]

Though the authors could not explain the results, this RCT spurred other researchers to find the cause: sulfisoxazole binds albumin and displaces bilirubin in neonates, leaving the bilirubin free to bind to brain tissue, causing kernicterus. As a result of this, investigations of drug affinity for albumin became commonplace.

In any case, medical trials utilizing RCT methodology are currently accepted as one of the most important types of evidence regarding medical therapies, and Silverman and Day deserve some credit for this. Both men contributed immensely to the academic renown of Babies Hospital during the McIntosh Era. Silverman quoted Day years later: "A student is someone who thinks otherwise- it is dangerous to treat this healthy state of mind." This original remark could just as easily have come from Silverman.

Though Andersen's role in the emergence of RCTs in pediatrics was mostly limited to her expertise in pathology, her participation in these three trials suggests a commitment to this new clinical research methodology: in spite of her ever-expanding research agenda, she recognized some value in this new methodology. Throughout her career, she possessed the ability to identify important new ideas that affected the practice of medicine.

Not to mention a seemingly endless capacity for work.

References

1. Silverman WA. Oral history project: William A. Sliverman, MD, L.M. Gartner, Editor. American Academy of Pediatrics; 1997.
2. Silverman WA. Personal reflections on lessons learned from randomized trials involving newborn infants from 1951 to 1967. Clin Trials. 2004;1(2):179–84.
3. Silverman WA. In search of the spirit of Babies Hospital. In: Babies Hospital, editor. Babies Hospital historical collection, 1887–1994. Archives at the Augustus C. Long Health Sciences Library of Columbia University.

4. Blodi FC, et al. Experiences with corticotrophin (ACTH) in the acute stage of retrolental fibroplasia. AMA Am J Dis Child. 1951;82(2):242–5.
5. Reese AB, et al. Results of use of corticotropin (ACTH) in treatment of retrolental fibroplasia. AMA Arch Ophthalmol. 1952;47(5):551–5.
6. Kinsey VE. Etiology of retrolental fibroplasia: preliminary report of a co-operative study of retrolental fibroplasia. Am J Ophthalmol. 1955;40(2):166–74.
7. Silverman WA, Andersen DH. Controlled clinical trial of effects of alevaire mist on premature infants. J Am Med Assoc. 1955;157(13):1093–6.
8. Silverman WA, Andersen DH. A controlled clinical trial of effects of water mist on obstructive respiratory signs, death rate and necropsy findings among premature infants. Pediatrics. 1956;17(1):1–10.
9. Silverman WA, et al. A difference in mortality rate and incidence of kernicterus among premature infants allotted to two prophylactic antibacterial regimens. Pediatrics. 1956;18(4):614–25.
10. Sinclair CJ. A difference in mortality rate and incidence of kernicterus among premature infants allotted to two prophylactic antibacterial regimens, by William A. Silverman, et al., Pediatrics, 1956;18:614-624. Pediatrics. 1998;102(1 Pt 2):225–7.

Babies Hospital Siblings

17

William Silverman noted that Babies Hospital "was an amazing place in 1944 and 1945. Names like Hattie Alexander and Jack Caffey and Beryl Paige, Mac McCune, one luminary after another" [1].

A decade later, Sidney Blumenthal was awed by the faculty members present at a routine, weekly conference:

> My first day at Babies was a Friday with, accordingly, attendance at the weekly Friday morning conference. I arrived early and took a seat in the middle of a rather drab amphitheatre. Dr. McIntosh arrived, sat in the center of the first row, and was soon surrounded by members of his staff. When the dust had settled, I took note. In the first few rows were Jack Caffey, Hattie Alexander, Dorothy Andersen, Virginia Apgar, Charley May, and Tom Santulli. And then Bill Silverman, Stan James, Mel Grumbach, Douglas Damrosch, Paul di Sant'Agnese, Ruth Harris, Bill Sansford, as well as Howard Mason, Katherine Merritt, Charley Wood, Harry Altman, and other distinguished clinicians… I was bewildered by this array of talent. Bewildered and subdued. Was this a special conference that had brought all these personalities together? No! This was a regular event. No attendance by edict. This was Rusty's family come to discuss and teach. Here they all were teachers first, clinicians, scientists, personalities. Siblings. [2]

Members of the Babies Hospital faculty during the McIntosh Era were occasionally better described as fractious siblings; however, they all shared an institutional pride in the advances in pediatric medicine made at their hospital.

It is notable that Dorothy Andersen collaborated on numerous "side" projects with many of her colleagues: some of these collaborations resulted in a published study, some did not. Brief sketches of several of these colleagues (or siblings) may help better understand the context of Andersen's career.

Like Andersen and Virginia Apgar, Hattie Alexander never married or had children. Her home near Long Island Sound was the center of several of her passions outside work, as described decades later toward the end of her career:

> Hattie lives in Port Washington, Long Island, with a physician friend, and commutes by train and subway, or by car… One of her chief joys is the greenhouse which she had built

J. S. Baird, *Dorothy Hansine Andersen*,
https://doi.org/10.1007/978-3-030-87484-1_17

into her home, and in which she indulges a longstanding hobby. Camellias have given way to less exotic plants, but she still cultivates a type of orchid … The speed boat in which she used to cruise the Sound has been sold. She particularly enjoys symphony recordings and hi-fi. [3]

Toward the end of the 1940s, Alexander began to focus more of her research efforts on microbial genetics in an attempt to better define the nature of genes. In 1950, Alexander and her assistant Grace Leidy reported using DNA to transform the capsular type of *Haemophilus influenzae* [4, 5], an important validation of the work by Oswald Avery's group on pneumococci several years earlier at the Rockefeller Institute. Alexander's interests then began to shift away from genetic transmission of information by bacteria toward its transmission by viruses, and using the most up-to-date lab technologies available, she suggested in 1958 that "the gene of polioviruses and other allied viruses is indeed a nucleic acid, not of the type found in bacteria and mammalian cells, DNA, but the variety found at that time, only in plants, ribonucleic acid (RNA)" [3]. Later in her career, she was the first woman to serve as President of the American Pediatric Society and continued to work at Babies Hospital until her death from cancer in 1968.

Virginia Apgar, like Andersen, began her career with an internship in surgery, but did not continue in that field. Following the advice of the Chair of the Department of Surgery at Columbia University, she began to study anesthesiology and eventually was Chief of the Division of Anesthesiology at CUMC before that division became a department. When Emanuel Papper was recruited to serve as the first Chair of the new Department of Anesthesiology in 1949, Apgar was relieved of many administrative tasks, and she then developed a focus on obstetric anesthesiology and subsequently on neonatology. In 1953 she published "A proposal for a new method of evaluation of the newborn infant"; institutional tradition suggests that she developed this score over breakfast.

> The story, often told at Columbia, is that a medical student on her service asked Dr. Apgar at breakfast how to evaluate a newborn. "That's easy, you would do it like this," said Virginia. She grabbed a napkin and jotted down 5 points, then rushed off to the obstetric unit to try it out. [6]

The easy-to-use Apgar score has been an important part of routine practice in the assessment of a neonate's condition ever since.

Apgar also worked with L. Stanley James to better define many of the clinical concerns related to neonatal asphyxia and resuscitation and with Richard Day on animal models of lung expansion during positive pressure ventilation. In 1959, Apgar retired from Babies Hospital and Columbia University and accepted an executive position with the March of Dimes:

> [She] devoted the rest of her life to fostering public support for research on birth defects. With missionary zeal, she traveled throughout the world, educating the public to the need for research into the prevention and treatment of birth defects and raising funds toward this end. Largely as a result of these efforts, the annual income of the National Foundation [of the March of Dimes] increased from $19 million when she arrived to $46 million at the time of her death. [7]

Apgar's interests outside of her academic and professional career were so numerous that many of her friends only knew of a few; this list is still incomplete: music, including proficiency with and manufacture of various stringed instruments; stamp collecting; sports, including tennis, golf, hiking, and both fly and deep sea fishing; fast cars, gardening, flying, and travel.

Neither Apgar nor Alexander ever collaborated with each other or with Andersen, and they were not close friends. Nevertheless, this trio of women physicians was the most successful and renowned group of all the Babies Hospital faculty from the McIntosh Era. They were each born in the first decade of the twentieth century, they shared several educational experiences (Andersen and Apgar both graduated from Mount Holyoke College, Andersen and Alexander both graduated from Johns Hopkins University's School of Medicine, and Andersen and Apgar both received training in surgery), and they were each successful in an academic career, all while they enjoyed living life by their own rules.

Frederic (Freddy) H. Bartlett was perhaps the most colorful character on the Babies Hospital faculty during the McIntosh Era (where the standards of eccentricity were quite high) as noted in a profile of him in *The New Yorker* in 1944:

> When a Long Island mother telephoned to ask how her chauffeur, who was to meet Dr. Bartlett at the local station, would be able to recognize him, he [Bartlett] told her, "If he sees somebody in a wrinkled suit, torn collar, and run-down shoes, with a battered hat and shaggy hair, somebody who looks like a dirty old bum, that'll be me." [8]

However, it wasn't just his appearance that caused a stir:

> Dr. Bartlett has what is known, to his dismay, as a *Social Register* practice, but, as he frequently says, his lack of tact has lost him enough rich patients to make up the most lucrative practice in town. He is an ardent and vocal enthusiast for a redistribution of wealth and for high taxes. [8]

Whatever his political interests, Bartlett had excellent clinical instincts: his comments in the Discussion section immediately following Dorothy Andersen's 1938 landmark CF study suggested that he quickly grasped the nature of this new disease. He was able to recognize several patients from his own practice who likely had CF and added:

> In summary: Cystic fibrosis of the pancreas is a nucleus about which is being crystallized a symptomatology. The condition should be considered a new clinical entity, and I feel that Dr. Andersen has contributed a great piece of work in that connection. [9]

A few years earlier, Bartlett had become quite popular when he published a book on childcare:

> When young parents speak of "Bartlett's," the chances are better than even that the book they mean is not "Familiar Quotations," by the late John Bartlett, but "Infants and Children: Their Feeding and Growth," by Frederic Huntington Bartlett, M.D., who, now seventy-two, is one of the hardest-working and best-known pediatricians in the city. [8]

To assume that Bartlett lacked academic inclinations would be a mistake: he coauthored several studies earlier in his career with Martha Wollstein (on brain tumors in young children [10] and on the incidence of tuberculosis in Babies Hospital autopsies [11]) and also published studies on topics as varied as high altitude pulmonary edema (then referred to as mountain sickness), infant dietary practices, polio, and streptococcal bacteremia following tonsillectomy.

Shortly after Andersen joined the Babies Hospital faculty in 1935, a friendship developed between Andersen and Hilde Bruch: Bruch was a German pediatrician who fled Nazi Germany in 1933 and was hired by McIntosh and mentored by Donovan McCune. McCune was the Director of Chemical Laboratories and the Chief of Clinic at the Vanderbilt Clinic. One of his colleagues – William Silverman – described McCune as "brilliant... he had a very incisive mind... he was a role model" [1]. McCune and Bruch explored the McCune-Albright syndrome [12], congenital hypothyroidism, and developmental changes in the adrenal glands. They seem an unlikely pair: Bruch, brilliant but burdened with family sorrows (her family was Jewish, and many of them were trapped in Germany during the war) and often frustrated with the vagaries of life in the United States, while McCune was an epicurean – his interests included winemaking, book publishing, and Latin.

In the late 1930s, Bruch began to investigate obesity in children, hypothesizing that the cause was likely related to metabolic or endocrine disease. Andersen offered statistical assistance [13], and in 1939 Bruch concluded that there was little or no evidence of metabolic or endocrine disorders in her obese patients [14, 15]. She then began to consider further training in psychiatry, and her own career reboot began in 1941: she left Babies Hospital to pursue psychiatric training at Johns Hopkins. She returned to CUMC in 1943 in the Department of Psychiatry, and her research was then focused on eating disorders for the remainder of her career. She remained a close friend of Andersen until Andersen's death.

John Caffey was another colorful character at Babies Hospital, though not perhaps in dress or politics: Silverman described Caffey as a "curmudgeon... He was very gruff... [but] was in many ways a role model" [1]; others agreed:

> He valued the life of the intellect highly, and he was well aware that he had been particularly blessed in mental acuity. He did not suffer fools gladly. At least at Babies Hospital, he taught in part by fear. [16]

It was Silverman who nicknamed him "Cactus Jack." Caffey's development as a pediatric radiologist early in his career at Babies Hospital was unusual and seems somewhat apocryphal:

> After one of these conferences [in which a pathologist discussed pediatric radiology findings], Dr. Caffey (who seldom minced words) remarked that it had been another hour wasted. He was overheard by the chief of pediatrics, who asked if he thought he could do better. His bluff called, Dr. Caffey replied to the effect that he could hardly do worse. He was forthwith put in charge of the hospital radiology department, and pediatric radiology became his life's work. [16]

In 1946 Caffey described a series of six infants with chronic subdural hematomas and multiple long bone fractures in the absence of a history of significant injury and without evidence of bone disease [17]. Caffey wrote: "In one of these cases the infant was clearly unwanted by both parents and this raised the question of intentional ill-treatment of the infant; the evidence was inadequate to prove or disprove this point" [17]. This early report helped introduce the difficult topic of nonaccidental trauma to pediatricians. Caffey published in 1941 one of the first textbooks on the utility of X-rays in children ("Roentgen Diagnosis in Infants and Children" [18]), expanded several years later as "Pediatric X-ray Diagnosis"; this textbook helped establish the subspecialty of pediatric radiology.

Caffey collaborated with Dorothy Andersen [19] and numerous other Babies Hospital colleagues on various studies in the 1950s. When Caffey was presented with the American Pediatric Society's Howland Award in 1965 from then-president Hattie Alexander, he said: "let me tell you Hattie Alexander, long-time friend and one-time colleague, that I am delighted to receive the Howland Medal and Award from your gracious hands, and this special treat makes the ceremony doubly precious" [20]. He was "perhaps the most eminent of the pioneers of pediatric radiology" [16].

Richard Day's career at Babies Hospital included collaborations with Dorothy Andersen, Virginia Apgar, Ruth Harris, Conrad Riley, and William Silverman, among others, but his main focus was the emerging field of neonatology. He helped design a new unit/ward to care for newborn babies at Babies Hospital [21] in the late 1940s which would eventually become one of the first Neonatal ICUs. He also played a critical role in the development of RCTs in pediatrics, as noted in the previous chapter. He left Babies Hospital in 1953 to become the Chair of Pediatrics at the State University of New York's Downstate Medical School and later served as Chair of Pediatrics at the University of Pittsburgh. He also received the Howland Award from the American Pediatric Society in 1986. Silverman described him as "the yeastiest character on the Babies Hospital staff … during the golden years of the McIntosh Era at Columbia" [21].

Melvin Grumbach completed a fellowship in pediatric endocrinology with Lawson Wilkins at Johns Hopkins and was the first Chief of Pediatric Endocrinology at Babies Hospital in 1955. His research work included over 300 publications, including in particular studies to help define hormonal control and dysfunction during growth and development, as well as the Barr body and the Lyon hypothesis, sexual differentiation, and congenital adrenal hyperplasia. He was "the world's foremost pediatric endocrinologist" according to his colleague, Walter Miller.

Beryl Paige (with Abner Wolf and David Cowen) was the first to show that *Toxoplasma gondii* could infect humans. The index case was an infant who died with seizures and chorioretinitis in June 1938. At autopsy, Paige noted encephalitis, hydrocephalus, and chorioretinitis, with multiple granulomas[1] and "a protozoan parasite, often in great numbers" [22] (Fig. 17.1).

---

[1] An area of inflammation often characterized by the presence of a particular cell type (macrophages) seen on microscopic examination.

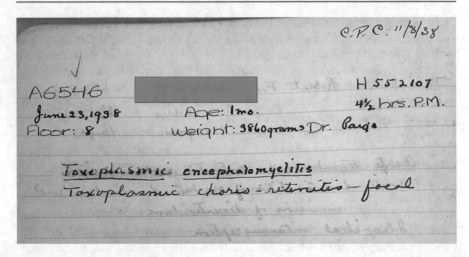

Fig. 17.1 The entry in the Babies Hospital autopsy register for the first patient with toxoplasmosis identified by Paige (she also appears to have signed her own name). (Photo by JS Baird, 2020)

Paige and her colleagues were then able to transmit this parasitic infection to rabbits and mice [22, 23]. She coauthored several more studies in the 1930s and 1940s which included recognition of the important clinical features of this infection [24], as well as evidence that the infection may begin during fetal life [25]: this was one of the earliest reports of vertical transmission of an infection from a mother to her fetus. The apparent lack of maternal infection in this devastating disease was at first puzzling, but Paige and her coworkers were eventually able to show evidence of latent maternal infection. It became clear that congenital infection with toxoplasmosis could even account for some cases of pediatric epilepsy and encephalopathy. As Rustin McIntosh noted years later: "she [Paige] really put human toxoplasmosis on the clinical map" [26].

Conrad Riley with Richard Day reported in 1949 a series of five children with a previously unknown syndrome: excessive sweating and salivation, with episodes of hypertension and patchy erythema, cyclic vomiting, as well as the absence of tears [27]. This constellation of findings suggested central autonomic dysfunction, and the Riley-Day syndrome is now known as familial dysautonomia, and a genetic defect has been identified.

William Silverman's experiences during the 1940s as a trainee led him to write an account of caring for patients during a polio outbreak in New York City in the summer of 1944 [28]. Several years later, he was interviewed about this experience and offered a bit more detail:

> On one particular night, this was late summer, it was before air conditioning, just steaming hot in New York. We had 2 deaths in the [Drinker] respirator, our spirits were low, our jaws were slack, and the nurses were putting on these Kenny packs, Sister Kenny packs for poliomyelitis, steaming caldrons of hot water, taking these wool pads to put on, the wards were just incredibly hot. And the nurses were gliding back and forth to the patients, wearing these long dresses; it looked like a scene out of Florence Nightingale in the Crimean War,

unbelievable. And at 3:00 a.m. in the middle of the night, our attending arrived to make rounds. Drunk, his tie tied perfectly, but not in front, in back. He was lucid, and very dignified, and matter-of-fact, and with flashlights we made rounds on this polio ward at 3:00 a.m. under these unbelievable conditions. Interesting enough, his theme, patient after patient, is, how do you know that the Kenny packs are doing any good? Fifty percent of these children get better without paralysis, and this method of treating polio has never been really evaluated. How do you know that you're not making them worse? I was so insulted by this, you know, it's unbelievable; here's this drunk who comes up and accuses us of maybe making our patients worse. As time went on, months and years later, I realized that this was probably the most important learning experience of my entire medical training career, including pediatric training, after graduation from medical school. It was quite something. And I think this summarized the whole experience at Babies Hospital. I was with a group of people who were willing to say "how do we know;" this was very different from my educational experience up to that time. [1]

Silverman later identified Donovan McCune as the attending physician in this episode [28]. Apparently an early morning visit from the attending physician at Babies Hospital was not uncommon, as was noted about Freddy Bartlett: "Doctors who have served as interns under him at the Babies' Hospital recall that he [Bartlett] used to drop in on them at one or two in the morning and talk about art, religion, or baseball until daybreak" [8].

After serving as the Director of the Babies Hospital NICU, Silverman was recruited to be the Chief of Neonatal Intensive Care at the Children's Hospital of San Francisco in 1968 and remained there until his retirement. He continued to publish and provide mentorship to physician trainees until his death in 2004. His career included over 200 publications and numerous honors. Understanding that the complexity of disease processes does not often yield to a reductionist approach, he was fond of pointing out that "when faced with Newton's problem to discover the source of gravity, the reductionist cuts open the apple and looks inside" [29].

Babies Hospital during the McIntosh Era provided an opportunity to excel for many pediatricians – including women – eager to advance the care of sick children. While the individual contributions of faculty members were responsible for much of the hospital's academic success, a collegial atmosphere in which a variety of viewpoints could be vigorously debated, collaborations were common, and synergy possible, served to advance the practice of pediatrics at CUMC.

References

1. Silverman WA. Oral history project: William A. Sliverman, MD, L.M. Gartner, Editor. American Academy of Pediatrics; 1997.
2. Straus J, Strauss L. Rusty McIntosh by some of the many who experienced the essence of his presence at Babies Hospital, 1931–1960. Babies Hospital Alumni Association; 1987.
3. Turner L. From C student to winning scientist. Goucher Alumnae Quarterly. 1962:18–20.
4. Alexander HE, Leidy G. Transformation of type specificity of Hemophilus influenzae. AMA Am J Dis Child. 1950;80(5):877–8.
5. Alexander HE, Leidy G. Determination of inherited traits of H. influenzae by desoxyribonucleic acid fractions isolated from type-specific cells. J Exp Med. 1951;93(4):345–59.

6. Butterfield PM. Foundations of pediatrics: Virginia Apgar (1909-1974). Adv Pediatr Infect Dis. 2012;59(1):1–7.
7. Sicherman B, Green CH. Notable American women: the modern period: a biographical dictionary. Cambridge, MA: The Belknap Press of Harvard University Press; 1980.
8. Gill B. Profiles: Emergencies, advice for. The New Yorker, July 15, 1944. p. 26–32.
9. Andersen DH. Cystic fibrosis of the pancreas and its relation to celiac disease: a clinical and pathologic study. Am J Dis Chil. 1938;56(2):344–99.
10. Wollstein M, Bartlett FH. Brain tumors in young children: a clinical and pathologic study. Am J Dis Child. 1923;25(4):257–83.
11. Wollstein M, Bartlett FH. A study of tuberculous lesions in infants and young children, based on post-mortem examinations. Am J Dis Child. 1914;VIII(5):362–76.
12. McCune DJ, Bruch H. Osteodystrophia fibrosa: report of a case in which the condition was combined with precocious puberty, pathologic pigmentation of the skin and hyperthyroidism, with a review of the literature. Am J Dis Child. 1937;54(4):806–48.
13. Bruch JH. Unlocking the Golden cage: an intimate biography of Hilde Bruch, M.D. Gürze Books; 1996.
14. Bruch H. Obesity in childhood: I. Physical growth and development of obese children. Am J Dis Child. 1939;58(3):457–84.
15. Bruch H. Obesity in childhood: II. Basal metabolism and serum cholesterol of obese children. Am J Dis Child. 1939;58(5):1001–22.
16. Griscom NT. John Caffey and his contributions to radiology. Radiology. 1995;194(2):513–8.
17. Caffey J. Multiple fractures in the long bones of infants suffering from chronic subdural hematoma. Am J Roentgenol Radium Ther. 1946;56(2):163–73.
18. Caffey J. Roentgen diagnosis in infants and children. Nelson; 1941.
19. Caffey J, Andersen DH. Metastatic embryonal rhabdomyosarcoma in the growing skelton; clinical, radiographic, and microscopic features. AMA J Dis Child. 1958;95(6):581–600.
20. Caffey J. Significance of the history in the diagnosis of traumatic injury to children: Howland Award Address. J Pediatr. 1965;67(5, Part 2):1008–14.
21. Silverman WA. Richard L. Day--the quintessential skeptical inquirer. Presentation of the Howland award 1986. Pediatr Res. 1986;20(10):1009–12.
22. Wolf A, Cowen D, Paige BH. Toxoplasmic encephalomyelitis: III. A new case of granulomatous encephalomyelitis due to a protozoon. Am J Pathol. 1939;15(6):657–694.11.
23. Wolf A, Cowen D, Paige B. Human toxoplasmosis: occurrence in infants as an encephalomyelitis verification by transmission to animals. Science. 1939;89(2306):226–7.
24. Cowen D, Wolf A, Paige BH. Toxoplasmic encephalomyelitis: VI. Clinical diagnosis of infantile or congenital toxoplasmosis; survival beyond infancy. Arch Neurol Psychiatr. 1942;48(5):689–739.
25. Wolf A, Cowen D, Paige BH. Fetal encephalomyelitis: prenatal inception of infantile toxoplasmosis. Science. 1941;93(2423):548–9.
26. Rustin McIntosh papers. Archives at the Augustus C. Long Health Sciences Library of Columbia University.
27. Riley CM, Day RL, et al. Central autonomic dysfunction with defective lacrimation; report of five cases. Pediatrics. 1949;3(4):468–78.
28. Silverman WA. In search of the spirit of Babies Hospital. In: Babies Hospital, editor. Babies Hospital historical collection, 1887–1994. Archives at the Augustus C. Long Health Sciences Library of Columbia University.
29. Silverman WA. Snobbery and gamesmanship in medical research. Paediatr Perinat Epidemiol. 2005;19(1):2–3.

A Last Decade of CF Research

Dorothy Andersen was named Chief of Pathology at Babies Hospital in 1952 after Beryl Paige retired for medical reasons [1]. Andersen was promoted to Associate Professor (of Pathology) in 1954, 19 years after beginning her career at Babies Hospital and 16 years after her landmark 1938 CF study. Following her landmark studies on CF heat prostration in 1951 and the first CF sweat study in January 1953, Andersen remained committed to CF research and improved CF care in spite of advancing age and numerous competing research interests. But her focus during her last decade of research in CF shifted from the early, fundamental questions, to include general (albeit detailed) reviews of CF, as well as attempts to answer a few of the many questions which emerged along with an increased awareness of that disease's multisystem nature.

At the same time an explosion of research and international interest in CF care occurred and was associated with the emergence of several new themes, including (but not limited to) improvements in diagnosis with sweat testing, *Pseudomonas* lung infections, the utility of chest physiotherapy and pulmonary function testing, cor pulmonale as a complication of chronic lung disease, and CF as a chronic disease in adults. Though Andersen was among the earliest to mention several of these themes (including sweat testing [2], *Pseudomonas* lung infections [3], cor pulmonale [4], and CF in adults [5]), there were many new names who began to dominate CF research during the 1950s, including Charlotte Anderson, Giulio Barbero, Robert Denton, LeRoy Matthews, and Archie Norman, among many others. Expertise in CF was no longer limited to New York City or Boston: by the end of the decade, the torch had been passed to a new generation.

Nevertheless, a review of Andersen's contributions during this time is helpful and may contribute to a better understanding of her concerns about the disease she helped define, as these were to be her final contributions to the study and care of CF. Though much of Andersen's research interests following the CF sweat studies of 1953 were focused on pediatric heart diseases, she clearly felt a duty to advise CF families regarding some of the important dietary, financial, educational, and social issues which she had identified over nearly two decades spent caring for patients with CF.

In 1955[1] Andersen coauthored a report on dietary problems and therapy in CF and celiac disease [6]. This report was of particular interest to parents, many of whom requested reprints, including those in the Washington D.C. chapter of the NCFRF:

> The Washington D.C. Chapter of the NCFRF includes the parents of celiac children as well as parents of [children with] CF … The parents often call particular articles to the attention of their attending pediatricians, also, as the doctors are bound to miss seeing some of the very articles in which they would be most interested. [7]

Dietary recommendations for CF in this report were similar to those made by Andersen a decade earlier [8]: the provision of an excess of calories using a low-fat and high-protein diet, vitamin supplementation, and the use of pancreatic enzymes. For celiac disease, gluten should be avoided. The authors also suggested that young children may benefit from frequent small feedings and that a "greater emphasis on restriction of fatty foods in pancreatic deficiency [CF] and on avoidance of starches in patients with celiac disease [6]" would be helpful. Parents were particularly happy to find specific meal plans for patients with these diseases at various ages in this report.

Andersen explored several of the most frustrating financial, educational, and social issues she knew patients and their families were facing in the late 1950s [9].[2] This report was unique in that it raised issues Andersen did not explore elsewhere and was published in a journal which was not widely available. Quoting a long section helps underscore some of the concerns for CF patients and their families that she felt deeply:

> These families need help of all kinds, financial, medical, educative, and supportive …
>
> First, the immediate care of the patient requires supervision by a doctor or clinic familiar with the disease, able to instruct the mother, and able to provide her with continued emotional support. At home the child needs daily vitamin supplements, salt tablets, and usually antibiotics of some sort. He does better on a planned diet, which the mother must learn how to prepare.
>
> The mother of the child with cystic fibrosis has many difficult decisions to make. Can Jim play with other children? Is isolation or exposure to infection the greater risk? How much exercise can the child stand? Will other mothers fear that his cough means a contagious disease? Shall he go to school or have home teaching? Can he go swimming? (The answer is yes.). How can his condition be explained to his grandparents and to the neighbors?
>
> The child himself, as he grows older, learns that he is different from other children. He may also learn that many children with cystic fibrosis die before they grow up. As he reaches adolescence he has new worries. What kind of work will he be able to do? Should he marry? How long a life should he plan for? With these problems added to the usual strains of adolescence, it is not surprising that some adolescents with this disease become deeply depressed.

---

[1] Originally presented at a meeting of the American Dietetic Association in 1954.

[2] Andersen actually presented this at a 1959 research meeting of the American Public Health Association, but it was not published until 1960.

The financial problems are staggering. Hospital bills are usually covered only in part by hospital insurance. Even if the child escapes hospitalization, the cost of his illness adds an estimated $1000 to $1500 a year in druggists' bills, X-rays, trips to the clinic, high protein foods with plenty of meat. Families of moderate income sometimes deprive the rest of the family of protein foods so that the sick child may have enough. Some sell their homes to pay the bills. Many parents who can see little improvement in their child from all the other measures they have taken decide to move their family to another climate, often at financial sacrifice and usually without benefit.

The genetic implications of the disease present other problems. The most pressing for the parents is often the question of whether or not to have more children. Shall they take a chance, and have other children of their own? Or shall they adopt a child, go in for artificial insemination, or perhaps get a divorce and begin over again? Sometimes the two sets of grandparents come into the conflict, each set convinced that the bad inheritance must come from the other.

Finally, many families feel isolated by what seems to them a unique problem, and many feel resentment because of the delay in diagnosis which resulted from their doctor's lack of knowledge about the disease. Many have been frustrated in their attempts to obtain assistance from public agencies to meet the heavy burden imposed on them by the disease. [9]

These were difficult questions that Andersen had confronted frequently; she suggested the need for more research, information dissemination to a wider audience, and an increase in public aid. The understanding and sympathy manifest in her comments shows why patients and their families loved her; her comments also reveal that her reputation for honesty was deserved.

Among the topics of the more pedestrian studies on CF she coauthored in the late 1950s were vitamin E deficiency in CF, medical care for adults with CF, and a decreased tendency to atherosclerosis in some patients with CF. As it was Andersen's final collaboration on CF with di Sant'Agnese, their investigation of the care of adults with CF deserves special comment.

The median survival for patients with CF increased at the same time that a spectrum of CF disease severity became apparent: more and more CF patients were identified who survived into adulthood, in part because some seemed to have a milder disease. Andersen and di Sant'Agnese investigated some of the problems which commonly affected adults with CF [5] and recognized this milder form in some adults, noting that "the majority of older patients have chronic bronchitis, generalized obstructive emphysema and chronic sinusitis. In rare individuals there is almost no pulmonary involvement at any time" [5]. Complications more frequently encountered in young adults with CF compared to children included sinusitis, hemoptysis, spontaneous pneumothorax, cirrhosis, abdominal masses,[3] and diabetes mellitus. Though their cohort of adult patients may have been small, their observations were astute.

They offered a case report in their 1959 study which seemed to support an improved probability of survival into adulthood for many patients with CF, including those with the most severe pulmonary disease, as long as a rigorous therapeutic course was followed [5]:

---

[3] This problem is now better known as diffuse intestinal obstruction syndrome.

C.J., a white male … was diagnosed … in 1940 at the age of 16 months … The patient was
kept on a diet low in fat and high in protein content, and pancreatic extracts were consistently given by mouth. He was virtually never off antibiotics ever since they became available and frequently received courses of intensive therapy with drugs administered by
intramuscular injection, by inhalation and by mouth. Despite this, through the years the
severity of the pulmonary involvement increased… during a relapse of the pulmonary
infection, he died rather suddenly. [5]

Though this patient died at 20 years of age and the clinical course was relentlessly
progressive, it was possible to glimpse some hope for the future in the narrative:
therapies directed at the major manifestations of CF in some patients were associated with an improved survival into childhood in the 1940s and 1950s, and into
adulthood in the 1950s and 1960s, and it was conceivable that further optimization
of CF therapies might lead to a normal lifespan for some CF patients. However,
there was clearly a price to pay for increased survival: for C.J., the price included
having to endure relentlessly progressive lung disease requiring frequent hospitalizations and included "many a tough year," as well as a shortened lifespan. The
courage and dedication of patients, families, and their medical teams were critical
to the improvement of medical care for CF in the twentieth century.

In 1962 Andersen published a review of the glandular pathology in CF [10]. The
discovery of the epithelial cell channelopathy responsible for CF was still several
decades in the future, and her review of problems involving obstruction or hyperse-
cretion of mucous glands as well as altered secretions from serous glands in CF
concluded with the suggestion that "This is a genetic disorder involving a variety of
cell types [10]" which affect exocrine gland secretions. She suggested several
hypotheses which might explain this, including whether the defect was "concerned
with the provision of energy for several types of secretion or whether it is more
directly related to control of secretion of electrolytes or of mucopolysaccharides"
[10]. More than half a century later the complex interplay of the CF channelopathy's
effect on the control of electrolyte secretion by epithelial cells and resultant organ
dysfunction remains an active field of investigation.

As lung function worsens in many patients with CF, similar to what occurs in
other chronic airway diseases, the heart is subjected to progressively increased
strain in order to send blood out to the lungs; this leads eventually to cor pulmonale
(failure of the right ventricle of the heart due to severe lung disease). The first mention of cor pulmonale in CF was by Andersen in 1949 [4]; it was a peripheral observation and she didn't present any data. However, it is easy to envision her deciding
to investigate this phenomenon further at some later date (she would have added it
to her list in 1949 after finishing her investigation of the vitamin A deficiency
hypothesis: one can envision that this list might include abnormal sweat and CF, cor
pulmonale and CF, *Pseudomonas* lung infection and CF, etc.). In 1951, one of the
earliest reports of cor pulmonale in CF described this condition in 25 young children with CF who died at Babies Hospital [11]: though this report included
Andersen's CF patients, Andersen was not an author nor was she acknowledged.
Interestingly, the author Stephen Royce (then a resident physician at Babies

Hospital[4]) did acknowledge the help of Rustin McIntosh, Richard Day, and John Caffey. Although lacking a pathophysiologic explanation, this retrospective study supported the idea that CF was frequently associated with cor pulmonale.

Toward the end of her career, Andersen worked on a major physiologic study of cor pulmonale in CF: the resulting posthumous publication in 1964 by a group of Columbia University internists and pediatricians (of which Andersen was the last or senior author) identified chronic hypoxia in the pathogenesis of pulmonary hypertension in CF [12]. They noted that pulmonary hypertension may lead to cor pulmonale and described 21 patients with CF who underwent cardiac catheterization and exposure to different inspired concentrations of oxygen, as well as spirometry and blood gas sampling: hypoxia was associated with an increase in pulmonary artery pressure which was reversible with oxygen therapy. As there was no apparent change in pulmonary blood flow during reversal of pulmonary hypertension, the authors reasoned that pulmonary vasoconstriction (associated with hypoxia) was responsible for CF-associated pulmonary hypertension and possibly with the eventual development of cor pulmonale in some CF patients. Had she lived, it is very likely that Andersen would have explored the possibility of chronic oxygen therapy in patients with more severe CF. This early study of pulmonary hypertension in CF has been cited more than a hundred times.

One of the potential topics in CF care that Andersen never got around to investigating was the utility of mechanical ventilation: as respiratory failure is common, especially late in CF, isn't mechanical support of breathing a valuable therapeutic option? With our current perspective decades later, the answer is "yes." We now have a variety of mechanical ventilation technologies to choose from: invasive vs noninvasive ventilators, including the capability to provide mechanical ventilation using either positive or negative pressure, and devices which provide high flow oxygen delivery, as well as many other support options. However this technology – and the intensive care units where this technology would first be utilized – began to emerge only at the end of Andersen's career. As Ruth Harris' case report on the care of tetanus [13] at Babies Hospital in the late 1940s demonstrated (Fig. 14.1), support of breathing (ventilation) at that time required ingenuity and persistence. Several early devices were available in some hospitals to assist ventilation in the 1950s: negative pressure ventilators (i.e., the Drinker respirator referred to by Silverman in his 1944 anecdote about polio in Babies Hospital) and cough-assist therapy to transiently inflate and deflate the lungs (using a device known as the "coughalator," developed by CUMC's brilliant pulmonologist Alvan Barach). These devices were utilized mostly for the victims of polio epidemics. Andersen was aware of these early technologies and used them, but her focus was not on mechanical ventilatory support in CF, as she noted:

---

[4] From a well-to-do southern California family, educated at Princeton and Harvard, and a young friend of Edwin Hubble, Royce returned to California following pediatric residency training where he continued his interest and support for both pediatrics and CF. Why he refused to recognize Andersen in this study is not known.

Physical aids to the removal of material from the bronchial tree, such as postural drainage and negative pressure, as in the "cough machine" [i.e., the coughalator] have been used, the results being variously reported. They are more effective in older children. [14]

It was only in 1978 long after Andersen's death that Pamela Davis and Paul di Sant'Agnese coauthored the first report on the use of mechanical ventilatory support in CF [15]. However, the retrospective, multicenter study by Davis and di Sant'Agnese documented a mostly dismal outcome for CF patients treated with positive pressure (invasive) mechanical ventilation. Improvement in the survival of CF patients treated with mechanical ventilation was noted decades later with the advent of lung transplantation and the availability of a broader range of ventilatory support technologies, as well as a better understanding of disease pathophysiology.

In 1958, 29 years after beginning her career in pathology at CUMC's Presbyterian Hospital and 23 years after moving to Babies Hospital, Andersen was promoted to Professor of Pathology at Columbia University's College of Physicians and Surgeons [16]; this promotion came two decades after her first landmark CF study. The academic rank of professor was then quite difficult for women to achieve; among her peers, Hattie Alexander, Virginia Apgar, and Hilde Bruch were recognized with that rank after 25, 12, and 25 years at Columbia University, respectively. By 1960, at least 600 patients with CF had been diagnosed and treated at Babies Hospital [17]: some had died, and some had moved away or returned to their home in another state as regional centers for CF care began to appear in many U.S. medical centers. Toward the end of Andersen's career in late 1962, there were about 200 active CF patients cared for in the Babies Hospital CF clinic [1].

Though she remained steadfastly dedicated to her CF patients and to her CF research efforts, she continued to develop new interests well into her third decade at Babies Hospital: between 1960 and her death in 1963, she authored or coauthored eleven studies, seven of which were investigations of pediatric heart diseases. These investigations strongly suggest an emerging research agenda she would have pursued more extensively if her life had not been cut short.

References

1. Presbyterian Hospital. Annual report of the Presbyterian Hospital in the City of New York. New York: The Presbyterian Hospital in the City of New York; 1939-64.
2. Darling RC, et al. Electrolyte abnormalities of the sweat in fibrocystic disease of the pancreas. Am J Med Sci. 1953;225(1):67–70.
3. Andersen DH. The present diagnosis and therapy of cystic fibrosis of the pancreas. Proc R Soc Med. 1949;42(1):25–32.
4. Andersen DH. Therapy and prognosis of fibrocystic disease of the pancreas. Pediatrics. 1949;3(4):406–17.
5. Di Sant'Agnese PA, Andersen DH. Cystic fibrosis of the pancreas in young adults. Ann Intern Med. 1959;50(5):1321–30.
6. Andersen DH, Mike EM. Diet therapy in the celiac syndrome. J Am Diet Assoc. 1955;31(4):340–6.

7. Dorothy H. Andersen papers. Archives at the Augustus C. Long Health Sciences Library of Columbia University.
8. Andersen DH. Celiac syndrome: III. Dietary therapy for congenital pancreatic deficiency. Am J Dis Child. 1945;70(2):100–13.
9. Andersen DH. Cystic fibrosis and family stress. Children. 1960;7(1):9–12.
10. Andersen DH. Pathology of cystic fibrosis. Ann N Y Acad Sci. 1962;93(12):500–17.
11. Royce SW. Cor pulmonale in infancy and early childhood; report on 34 patients, with special reference to the occurrence of pulmonary heart disease in cystic fibrosis of the pancreas. Pediatrics. 1951;8(2):255–74.
12. Goldring RM, et al. Pulmonary hypertension and cor pulmonale in cystic fibrosis of the pancreas. J Pediatr. 1964;65:501–24.
13. Harris RC, McDermott TR, Montreuil FL. The treatment of tetanus. Pediatrics. 1948;2(2):175–85.
14. Andersen DH. Cystic fibrosis of the pancreas. J Chronic Dis. 1958;7(1):58–90.
15. Davis PB, di Sant'Agnese PA. Assisted ventilation for patients with cystic fibrosis. JAMA. 1978;239(18):1851–4.
16. Sicherman B, Green CH. Notable American women: the modern period: a biographical dictionary. Cambridge, MA: The Belknap Press of Harvard University Press; 1980.
17. Doershuk CF. Cystic fibrosis in the 20th century: people, events, and progress. Cleveland: AM Publishing Ltd; 2001.

Pediatric Heart Diseases

19

As recently noted, "It is historically important to realize that in the early years of the 20th century, every child born with a congenital heart defect was destined to succumb to its effects, the only variable was timing; either hours or a handful of years" [1]. This was the context in which Dorothy Andersen began her career in pediatric pathology, and it helps explain her blossoming interest in pediatric cardiology as surgical and other therapeutic options began to emerge in the middle of the twentieth century.

In spite of increased responsibilities as Babies Hospital's chief pathologist, Andersen continued to pursue numerous side projects in addition to her work on CF, celiac disease, and glycogen storage diseases. As opposed to her colleague Hattie Alexander's systematic investigations in microbiology, which arose from sequentially posing questions whose answers would advance biologic knowledge incrementally, Andersen was always searching in a variety of new directions – often simultaneously – with the hope of making insightful, if unsuspected, discoveries. She realized that many diseases were poorly defined (and likely represented syndromes) and that a rigorous investigation of these syndromes might yield unexpected results; that was the case with celiac syndrome as well as with glycogen storage diseases. Though numerous pediatric heart diseases were already well-defined by the 1950s, she wondered if there might be some common pathophysiologic mechanisms in several of these diseases (e.g., heart failure or cyanosis) that might be addressed therapeutically; she became convinced that effective medical and surgical therapies for infants and children with congenital heart defects were not far off.

In a symposium on pediatric cardiology sponsored by the American Academy of Pediatrics in 1963, Sidney Blumenthal[1] suggested that:

---

[1] Blumenthal was recruited from Mount Sinai Hospital in New York City to join Babies Hospital as the Director of the Pediatric Cardiac Clinic in 1955. In 1960 he was promoted to Professor of Clinical Pediatrics at Columbia University's College of Physicians and Surgeons. After establishing and serving as the first Director of the Division of Pediatric Cardiology at Babies Hospital,

J. S. Baird, *Dorothy Hansine Andersen*,
https://doi.org/10.1007/978-3-030-87484-1_19

the contributions of Maude Abbott, Dorothy Andersen, and our own Helen Taussig need no recapitulation to this audience. I would in this regard like to emphasize the point that their monumental contributions were for the most part the result of the efforts of individuals working as individual investigators. [2]

Andersen and Blumenthal collaborated at Babies Hospital until Andersen's death a few months prior to this symposium, and Blumenthal's inclusion of Andersen with Abbott and Taussig reflected in part the grief he felt at the recent loss of his colleague and collaborator. Recognition of Andersen as a pioneer in pediatric cardiology was not common beyond the confines of Columbia University.

Female physicians have been closely linked to the development of pediatric cardiology, including in particular Maude Abbott and Helen Taussig. Both were instrumental in the development of specific surgical interventions for congenital heart disease, though their importance to the development of pediatric cardiology is only partly related to these interventions. Abbott was educated in Canada and for much of her career was on the faculty of McGill University. She became interested in the persistence of a ductus arteriosus[2] in some infants: this abnormality is associated with increased pulmonary blood flow and may be occasionally life-threatening. Her interest was an important factor in the first surgical closure of a ductus arteriosus in 1938 [3].[3] Taussig graduated from Hopkins medical school in 1927 one year after Andersen and three years before Alexander. Taussig helped develop a shunt for cyanotic congenital heart diseases now known as the Blalock-Thomas-Taussig shunt: the subclavian artery is attached to the pulmonary artery, leading to increased pulmonary blood flow similar to the effect of having a persistent ductus arteriosus. An increase in pulmonary blood flow may decrease the cyanosis associated with some congenital heart malformations. The first Blalock-Thomas-Taussig shunt (in a human) was created in 1944 in a child with tetralogy of Fallot. Procedures to close or open various shunts were critically important in the growth of pediatric cardiology, as they offered the possibility of surgical palliation for a variety of congenital heart defects. While these palliative procedures did not always offer a definitive cure, they might be helpful in prolonging life until a complete repair was possible.

Though the contributions of Abbott and Taussig are well-known, Andersen's contributions to the emerging field of pediatric cardiology are not: a recent history of pediatric cardiology did not mention her [4], and most of the references to her efforts in this field are only to be found in sources closely related to Columbia University and/or Babies Hospital. It is difficult to be as enthusiastic about Andersen's contributions to this field as was Blumenthal without more evidence.

Blumenthal later served as the Director of the Heart and Vascular Disease Division at the National Institute of Health.

[2] A blood vessel which connects the main pulmonary artery to the aorta, allowing blood from the right ventricle of the heart to bypass the lungs of a fetus (before birth the lungs do not participate in gas exchange). The ductus arteriosus usually closes within a few weeks of birth.

[3] Additional palliative procedures available during Andersen's lifetime to diminish pulmonary blood flow included the use of surgery or constrictive bands to narrow the pulmonary arteries, first described in 1952 by Muller and Dammann.

Andersen's contributions include studies of a variety of pediatric heart diseases, as well as direction and guidance of seminars and training sessions. The studies which she completed include descriptions of specific types of congenital heart disease [5–10], investigations of heart disease associated with CF [11, 12], and investigations of syndromes [13–16] and miscellaneous diseases of the heart [17, 18]. Documentation of any of the seminars and training sessions attributed to her is mostly unavailable. In addition, some of the work which she and Blumenthal envisioned was never completed, in large part due to Andersen's illness and untimely death. Evidence of her contributions to the development of pediatric cardiology are not easy to locate.

In 1956, Rustin McIntosh included in his annual report to the CUMC information about advances in pediatric cardiology during that year:

> With the close collaboration of the staff of pediatric radiology, Dr. Sidney Blumenthal and Dr. Dorothy H. Andersen organized a series of seminars on congenital malformations of the heart. These have not only attracted considerable attention but have also provided a better understanding of the potentialities for corrective surgery in conditions once regarded as beyond repair… The effect of all of these activities has been a greatly augmented interest on the part of the entire professional staff in the field of cardiology, and a considerably more aggressive and imaginative attack on clinical problems. [19]

Reference to Andersen's role in pediatric cardiology seminars over a decade earlier was also suggested in a biographical sketch of Andersen:

> During World War II surgeons pioneering in open-heart surgery, whose knowledge of cardiac embryology and anatomy was limited, sought Andersen's assistance. Asked to develop a training program, she did so, using her collection of congenital cardiac defects as illustrations. [20]

Douglas Damrosch offered a bit more detail about the seminars and training sessions:

> she [Andersen] conducted courses in the embryology and anatomy of cardiovascular abnormalities, and these sessions contributed materially to the training of those who were to be responsible for the development of open-heart surgery in the New York area. In addition she conducted seminars for the Babies Hospital staff through which a more and more physiologic approach to cardiac abnormalities was developed. [21]

Joshua Sonett, chief of general thoracic surgery at CUMC in 2019, emphasized the importance of Andersen's "collection of congenital heart defects":

> She [Andersen] would study the hearts of deceased pediatric patients and try to understand their defects. By keeping the specimens labeled and categorized, she integrated her basic studies of why children die with these bad hearts into the training programs of the surgeons at the time, so that they could see what the defects were and start to understand how to fix them at a time when cardiac surgery was in its infancy. [22]

Several of the autopsy specimens Andersen preserved are still to be found in the subbasement of Babies Hospital (now Morgan Stanley Children's Hospital of NewYork-Presbyterian) (Fig. 19.1).

Fig. 19.1 (**a**) Several of Dorothy Andersen's preserved autopsy specimens at Babies Hospital (including patients with 1. ventricular septal defect and dextraposition of the aorta, 2. patent ductus arteriosus, 3. pulmonary atresia with patent foramen ovale, 4. bicuspid pulmonary valve with ventricular septal defect and patent ductus arteriosus, 5. patent foramen ovale with ventricular septal defect and patent ductus arteriosus, and 6. esophageal atresia with tracheoesophageal fistula). (**b**) One of Andersen's preserved heart specimens with a probe passed through the patent ductus arteriosus. (Photos by JS Baird, 2020)

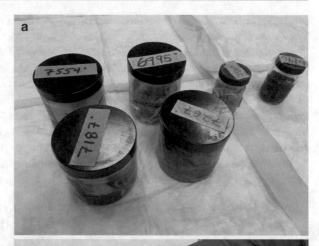

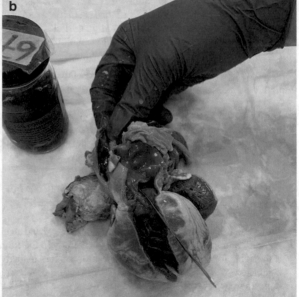

However, there is no evidence of Andersen's seminars or training programs in the CUMC Archives. It appears that Andersen viewed her publications as her legacy; she left very little evidence of her lectures, or early drafts of her publications, or the development of her thoughts on a particular topic. For Andersen, only the end result counted: scientific truth is reflected solely in its applicability to the gradual advance of science. In the twentieth century and currently, scientific truth is mostly limited to publication in peer-reviewed journals. Lectures and early drafts of a study are unlikely to contribute much, she must have felt, in that narrow context. While Hattie Alexander's CUMC Archives include the texts of numerous lectures and early drafts of studies, as well as material related to studies she never completed, this is not true for Andersen's CUMC Archives. Andersen apparently did not believe that the supporting evidence of lectures or early drafts or incomplete studies was important to preserve or that these might be of interest to future generations; in some ways, her self-deprecatory attitude encompassed both her private life and her professional career.

In the absence of any documentation of Andersen's participation in seminars and training programs for cardiac surgeons, it is difficult to determine the broad outlines for what she attempted to accomplish in pediatric cardiology: however, her collaborations with Blumenthal offer some hints.

In 1959, Blumenthal and Andersen described the results of three hundred and forty autopsies of infants and children with major cardiac malformations, as well as the clinical course of one hundred infants with heart failure, including results from cardiac catheterization, surgery, or autopsy, whenever available [16]. They concluded that most children with heart failure in infancy had acyanotic congenital cardiac malformations associated with increased pulmonary blood flow. Many of the patients with cyanotic congenital cardiac malformations had decreased pulmonary blood flow in the absence of heart failure symptoms. In any case, two thirds of infants with heart failure did not survive. The potential of altering pulmonary blood flow to improve survival of infants with heart failure was clearly something they were considering.

Two years later, their cohort of autopsies had grown to include four hundred and twenty-six autopsies of infants and children with major cardiac malformations, and Blumenthal and Andersen prepared an abstract for the American Heart Association's 1961 meeting. This abstract offers a small window into their shared concerns about developing treatments for congenital heart defects in infants:

> More patients succumb to the effects of congenital malformations of the heart during the first year of life than at any comparable period.... The findings in 426 autopsies, in which major congenital cardiac malformations were present, have been analyzed. Infants less than 1 year of age accounted for 75% (320) of the total. The hypoplastic left heart syndrome, a common cause of death in the first month, was infrequently noted later in infancy. Anomalies resulting in marked increase in pulmonary blood flow, although a frequent cause of death in the first month, increased in frequency still further in the 1- to 6-month period. A high proportion of anomalies encountered were considered to be amenable to palliative or corrective surgery. [5]

It was clear to Blumenthal and Andersen that the emerging field of pediatric cardiac surgery would need to focus mainly on infants. As definitive repair for the vast majority of congenital heart defects was not yet practical, they considered palliative interventions: could these interventions increase (like a Blalock-Thomas-Taussig shunt) or decrease (like closing a ductus arteriosus or applying a constrictive band to pulmonary arteries) pulmonary blood flow selectively and thus improve short-term survival? Definitive repair would require the refinement of technologies capable of supporting infants during heart surgery, including cardiopulmonary bypass (in which a mechanical device collects venous blood from a patient, decreases carbon dioxide and increases oxygen in that blood, and then pumps that blood back out via the aorta), cardioplegia (in which the heart's contractions are stopped in order to facilitate surgical interventions), manipulation of vasomotor tone (so that blood vessels in the lungs or the rest of the body dilate or contract as needed), and a variety of additional technologic interventions (antithrombosis, control of the heart rhythm, echocardiography, and therapeutic hypothermia among others); many of these technologies were not available for at least several years (or even decades) following Andersen's death. It is likely that Andersen's time commitments and illness prevented further work on this project; in any event, a larger study of this cohort was never published.

Andersen likely took a similar approach in seminars or training programs on congenital heart defects. Her experience at dissection would likely have given her some insight into the possible utility and complexity of various palliative procedures in particular patients, and her knowledge of physiology would have contributed to the practical application of these procedures.

As reviewed in an earlier chapter, toward the end of her life, Andersen helped investigate the role of hypoxia in the development of increased pulmonary vascular resistance in CF using cardiac catheterization[4] data from CF patients. Andersen must have considered the need for this kind of data to better define the problem of pulmonary blood flow in association with congenital heart disease, though the technology was still in its infancy. Andersen's work with Blumenthal suggests that therapeutic manipulation of abnormal pulmonary blood flow was a question she would have liked to investigate further – along with the use of emerging therapies for congenital heart defects – if cancer had not cut short her life.

It was not until the successful development and refinement of cardiopulmonary bypass that surgical repair of many complex congenital heart defects in infants became possible. Almost a decade after Blumenthal and Andersen presented their findings to the American Heart Association, and seven years after Andersen's death, Blumenthal collaborated with several pediatric cardiac surgeons to present data on the first fifteen open heart operations on infants utilizing cardiopulmonary bypass at Babies Hospital [23]: it then became possible to envision repairs on some of the most severe congenital heart defects.

Andersen would have been happy to hear of this and likely quick to minimize her own role in the development of pediatric cardiology as a subspecialty. Unfortunately, there is not enough evidence available to agree or disagree with that assessment. Her legacy is nonetheless impressive and consists of over a dozen published studies, many of them completed in the last few years of her life; it is likely that she envisioned much more.

---

[4] Andre Cournand and Dickinson Richards at Columbia University contributed to the development of cardiac catheterization and earned a share of the Nobel Prize in Medicine or Physiology in 1956.

References

1. Checchia PA, et al. The evolution of pediatric cardiac critical care. Crit Care Med. 2021;49(4):545–57.
2. Griffiths SP, Blumenthal S. A symposium: recent advances in cardiology. INTRODUCTION. Pediatrics. 1964;33(6):988–9.
3. Gross RE, Hubbard JP. Surgical ligation of a patent ductus arteriosus: report of first successful case. JAMA. 1984;251(9):1201–2.
4. Neill CA, Clark EB, Clark EP. The developing heart: a 'history' of pediatric cardiology. Springer; 1995.
5. Blumenthal S, et al. Congenital malformations of the heart in early infancy. Circulation. 1961;24(4):890.
6. Ellis K, et al. Congenitally corrected transposition of the great vessels. Radiology. 1962;79:35–50.
7. Griffiths SP, Levine OR, Andersen DH. Aortic origin of the right pulmonary artery. Circulation. 1962;25:73–84.
8. Jacobson JH 2nd, et al. Aberrant left pulmonary artery. A correctable cause of respiratory obstruction. J Thorac Cardiovasc Surg. 1960;39:602–12.
9. Kauffman SL, Andersen DH. Persistent venous valves, maldevelopment of the right heart, and coronary artery-ventricular communications. Am Heart J. 1963;66(5):664–9.
10. Kauffman SL, Ores CN, Andersen DH. Two cases of total anomalous pulmonary venous return of the supracardiac type with stenosis simulating infradiaphragmatic drainage. Circulation. 1962;25:376–82.
11. Goldring RM, et al. Pulmonary hypertension and cor pulmonale in cystic fibrosis of the pancreas. J Pediatr. 1964;65:501–24.
12. Holman RL, Blanc WA, Andersen DH. Decreased aortic atherosclerosis in cystic fibrosis of the pancreas. Pediatrics. 1959;24(1):34–9.
13. Andersen DH, Kelly J. Congenital endocardial fibro-elastosis. II. A clinical and pathologic investigation of those cases without associated cardiac malformations including report of two familial instances. Pediatrics. 1956;18(4):539–55.
14. Andersen DH, Kelly J. Endocardial fibro-elastosis. I. Endocardial fibro-elastosis associated with congenital malformations of the heart. Pediatrics. 1956;18(4):513–38.
15. Bailey FR, Andersen DH. Acute interstitial myocarditis. Am Heart J. 1931;6(3):338–48.
16. Blumenthal S, Andersen DH. Congestive heart failure in children. J Chronic Dis. 1959;9(5):590–601.
17. Di Sant'Agnese PA, et al. Glycogen storage disease of the heart. I. Report of 2 cases in siblings with chemical and pathologic studies. Pediatrics. 1950;6(3):402–24.
18. Di Sant'Agnese PA, Andersen DH, Mason HH. Glycogen storage disease of the heart. II. Critical review of the literature. Pediatrics. 1950;6(4):607–24.
19. Presbyterian Hospital. Annual report of the Presbyterian Hospital in the City of New York. New York: The Presbyterian Hospital in the City of New York; 1939-64.
20. Sicherman B, Green CH. Notable American women: the modern period: a biographical dictionary. Cambridge, MA: The Belknap Press of Harvard University Press; 1980.
21. Damrosch DS. Dorothy Hansine Andersen. J Pediatr. 1964;65:477–9.
22. It happened here: Dr. Dorothy H. Andersen. Health matters: stories of science, care & wellness. March 23, 2020. Available from: https://healthmatters.nyp.org/it-happened-here-dr-dorothy-h-andersen/.
23. Malm JR, et al. Open heart surgery in the infant. Am J Surg. 1970;119(5):613–6.

Part III

Beyond Babies Hospital and the McIntosh Era

When asked if he [Thoreau] had made his peace with God, he replied: "I did not know we had ever quarreled."
    Simon Critchley, The Book of Dead Philosophers.

As Dorothy Andersen's fame spread beyond Babies Hospital and New York City, she became an accepted authority on CF for physicians, patients, and their families around the world. By the beginning of her third decade at Babies Hospital and with the continued growth of her academic interests, she began to realize that it was also time to enjoy the view, to make the most out of whatever time remained to her. Though Babies Hospital remained at the center of her academic life, the growth of CF support organizations took up much of her time and energy, and Rustin McIntosh's retirement, as well as her own illness distanced her from the Babies Hospital that she knew.

Andersen, like many women physicians of her generation who pursued academic careers, never married and was childless. She was proud of her career and content with her choices in life, but she was well aware of the sacrifices she had made. The deaths of both her parents while she was a teenager, the tragic nature of CF for many of the infants and children she tried to help, and her own metastatic lung cancer, all contributed to her understanding of the fragile nature of life. While it is tempting to speculate about her religious inclinations (particularly in the context of her father's close connections to an organization with evangelical Christian roots), she left very little evidence of her feelings in that regard, or of her feelings about the sacrifices and losses she endured. In essence, she was a humanist, similar to her father: deeply concerned with offering dignity and support and care to individuals while she advanced the boundaries of medical knowledge for everyone.

In any event, she refused to let concerns about her sacrifices or losses, or even her illness, prevent her from enjoying life. She continued to spend time at her farm in northwest New Jersey, she enjoyed immensely her European trips, and she found novel ways to celebrate winter holidays. And she was always happy to share her enjoyment with others. Perhaps just as important, it appears that many of the qualities ascribed to her father—loyalty, candor, and honesty—could be used to describe her, even as she confronted her own mortality.

Time to Enjoy the View   20

By mid-1952, Dorothy Andersen was 51 years old, the age at which both of her parents had died. While she had no reason to expect that her life would also be cut short and that this would be her last decade, she did seem to become more aware that her productivity was limited by time. As a result, the range of her research interests increased without any slowing of her research output. She also began to smoke more as she contemplated the new research projects she hoped to pursue, including, as already noted, pediatric heart diseases.

She continued to have numerous interests outside of her medical research, and some of these seemed to recall her childhood and college career: bird-watching, hiking, and a variety of outdoor sports, all animated by a profound concern for the natural world. Other interests suggested her rural roots, as well as a love for doing work by hand: carpentry and construction, cooking on a wood stove, and gardening and harvesting food. Still other interests were a reflection of her profound intelligence and appreciation of other cultures: travel, foreign language skills, and a voracious appetite for reading.[1]

Andersen by then had enjoyed a successful career in academic medicine and was Chief of Pathology at Babies Hospital; she could not be faulted for focusing a bit more on some of her non-academic interests. Did she begin to wonder how best to spend the time remaining to her, how best to enjoy the view? No direct evidence exists to suggest this; however, late in 1952 Andersen moved from Manhattan's Washington Heights neighborhood to a house in Leonia, New Jersey [1]. Though it was only a short commute across the George Washington Bridge to CUMC from this more affluent suburban neighborhood, her move was a recognition of her decreased need for a home next-door to her workplace. After several decades, she reclaimed many of the possessions that she and her mother had placed in storage

---

[1] An example of the broad range of books which attracted Andersen was included in her response to an alumni questionnaire from Mount Holyoke College in 1960 about books she had read recently: *New Light on the Most Ancient East* by V. Gordon Childe, *Advise and Consent* by Allen Drury, and *The Mustard Seed Garden Manual of Painting* by Mai Mai Sze.

J. S. Baird, *Dorothy Hansine Andersen*,
https://doi.org/10.1007/978-3-030-87484-1_20

when they moved to Vermont from Summit decades earlier [2]. The photos and books, as well as any mementos that remained, would have been bittersweet reminders of the losses she had suffered, but also of the qualities she most admired in her parents, as well as of some of her favorite childhood memories.

Andersen was beginning to envision more of a life outside of work. Her new home in Leonia reminded her of her childhood in another affluent New Jersey suburb not too far away: Summit. It was, at least, a bit closer to her beloved farm. She had good friends in or near Leonia, among them, Marion Beman Chute, her classmate from Mount Holyoke College. And by late 1959 or early 1960, Andersen had another friend in Leonia, Celia Ores, who in 1960 began residency training in Pathology at CUMC [3].[2] Ores was mentored by Andersen and became a close friend, in spite of an age difference of nearly three decades. Ores remembered that Andersen was quite popular in Leonia: many of her friends there had no connection to her professional life [4].[3]

Douglas Damrosch suggested of Andersen during this time: "her hospitality was unbounded and literally scores of friends shared her home at one time or another. She freely offered her friendship; her loyalty to friends was unquestioned" [5]. Whether at work, or in Leonia, or at her farm, Andersen's dedication and concern for her colleagues and friends was widely recognized:

- At work, Henry Dunn, a new fellow at Babies Hospital, offered evidence of Andersen's hospitality:

  I arrived in New York by boat from England on 25 June 1952, to take up an appointment as Holt Fellow in Pediatrics and Assistant Pathologist attached to Drs. Beryl Paige and Dorothy Andersen at the Babies Hospital for one year. After a few hours in sweltering heat and humidity, I got through Customs with most of my worldly belongings, and I was amazed to find Dr. Dorothy Andersen waiting for me with her van at the dockside. This courtesy towards a Junior Assistant arriving from overseas impressed me greatly.... Dr. McIntosh came to the laboratory and Dr. Andersen introduced him to me... While trying to learn pediatric pathology I was impressed by the close linkage between clinicians and pathologists at the Babies Hospital.... Dr. Andersen conducted Ward Rounds, particularly on patients with malabsorption, and she even had an out-patient session for them. [6]

- In Leonia on Andersen's first visit to Ores' new home, Andersen asked Ores if she liked the wallpaper: Ores' negative response spurred Andersen to spend the rest of the afternoon removing wallpaper – and teaching Ores how to do it [4]. Ores suggested that similar episodes, in which Andersen offered help and hospitality to her many friends in Leonia, were common.

---

[2] Ores graduated from medical school in Bern, Switzerland, but was skeptical that anyone in the United States would hire her as she was "Polish, Jewish, and a refugee." Her early choice of training in pathology and later choice of a career in pediatrics was deeply influenced by Andersen.

[3] Andersen's CUMC Archives includes a note to Columbia University's Dean of Medicine after Andersen's death: "Leonia, New Jersey; March 12; Dr. Dorothy Andersen's close friends, nonmedical, wish to express their appreciation of the flowers sent by the Faculty of Medicine."

Fig. 20.1 Dorothy
Andersen as "Brew
Mistress" mixing glug in
her 8th floor lab at Babies
Hospital. (Courtesy of the
Journal of Pediatrics)

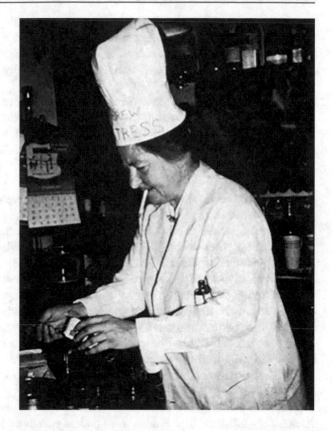

- At Andersen's farm, many physicians-in-training (including Michael Katz and
  Celia Ores during the last few years of Andersen's life[4]) were her guests, and
  celebrations with them usually included a memorable meal prepared by Andersen
  on her wood-burning stove [4], resulting in "weekends to remember" [5].

One way in which Andersen began to relax and enjoy the view even while she
was hard at work was to become a routine holiday celebration each winter at Babies
Hospital: Andersen's glug (Fig. 20.1).[5]

Glug (or glogg, a Scandinavian type of mulled wine) as Andersen mixed it
included "burgundy, cognac, cinnamon, cloves, and Thor knows what else" [5]: it
was powerful stuff, and physicians-in-training knew better than to drink too much.
Andersen deeply enjoyed this holiday tradition of her own making. In the last few

---

[4] Though Bijal Trivedi suggested in *Breath from Salt* that Paul di Sant'Agnese visited the farm with
his family, it is difficult to envision him enduring the primitive rural conditions voluntarily and
without complaint. Likewise it is difficult to envision Rustin McIntosh visiting Andersen's farm,
an event which Katz suggested was unlikely.

[5] Libby Machol suggested that glug – including the recipe – was an Andersen family tradition
which they brought from Bornholm.

years of her career, Michael Katz remembered her smoking cigarettes as she mixed the glug, the ash falling frequently into it. He pointed this out to her and asked if the ashes were important in the recipe: she laughed [7]. The glug was destined for consumption by all who worked at Babies Hospital, usually as part of a celebration around the Christmas season.[6]

As the "Brew Mistress" Andersen was quite willing to poke fun at herself: she refused to take herself too seriously, and she was mostly unafraid of what others might think of her choices. Though other faculty members might inspire anxiety or even fear, Andersen did not: she was less concerned with appearances and social expectations for women, usually willing to challenge the powerful, and always interesting.

Meeting Andersen as a student or physician-in-training was likely to have been a pleasant experience, as long as one was able to ignore the cigarette smoke. She was a renowned teacher, and students remembered her lectures with fondness: she "made a lasting impression" [8], and students felt "privileged to hear Dr. Dorothy Andersen present her description of this new disease" [8]. She was not reclusive or introverted and didn't appear to be lonely: rather she "freely offered her friendship" and had "scores of friends" [5], many of whom were younger physicians-in-training. She wasn't overbearing or intimidating, and a careful, rational approach characterized her interactions: "her modesty made her slow to advise, though her advice was always worth having" [5]. She didn't bully others into accepting the conclusions of her research, suggesting instead that "It is a matter worth considering, at any rate" [9]. Andersen was one of the most popular – and highly esteemed – faculty members at Babies Hospital in the McIntosh Era.

Andersen's example – and that of some of her women colleagues, like Hattie Alexander – affirmed that women were no less valuable than men in their competitive profession, and they both served as role models for the next generation of women in academic medicine: Andersen with less concern for fashion or for contemporary feminine standards of dress and Alexander with pearls and a definite sense of style, but both of them dedicated and eminently successful women who left important legacies (Fig. 20.2).

When the stress and strain of her work became a bit much and Andersen needed more of an escape than just a weekend at her farm, there was still another diversion that beckoned, another way that she could enjoy the view.

Always fond of trips to Europe since her extended tour in 1928 and 1929 following her surgery internship, she travelled there for more than just a few weeks in 1948, 1950, 1954, and 1956. Indirect evidence of several of these trips include her presence at conferences or hospital visits; it is quite possible that additional trips went undocumented. Her education and background, including familiarity with several foreign languages, suggest that cultural interests contributed to these excursions: she certainly shared with her own parents a broad knowledge of European

---

[6]There was, perhaps, one person at Babies Hospital who might not have approved of Andersen's glug: Rustin McIntosh. McIntosh's conservative nature might have made him uncomfortable with this event and could have contributed to a slightly strained relationship.

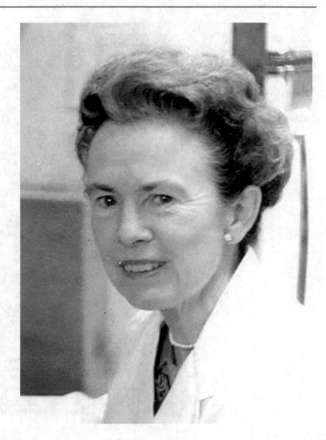

Fig. 20.2 Hattie Alexander. (Courtesy of the US National Library of Medicine)

culture and interests. She also profited from these occasions to visit friends, colleagues, and former trainees, like Winifred Young and Beryl Corner.

In the 1940s, Young, a pediatrician in England, was awarded a fellowship which allowed her to work with Andersen at Babies Hospital. She developed an interest in CF, a career in medical research,[7] as well as a lifelong friendship with Andersen. Corner, another English pediatrician who helped establish the subspecialty of neonatology in England,[8] also became a close friend and was an occasional guest at Andersen's farm whenever she visited the United States. During the 1950s, Young worked at the Queen Elizabeth Hospital for Children in London, and Corner worked at the Bristol Royal Hospital for Children in Bristol (Fig. 20.3).

Andersen's 1956 sabbatical in England was a singular event: an extended visit lasting 6 months; it gave her the freedom to discuss her work in a more relaxed manner with her British colleagues. In 1948 she had given lectures and participated in numerous discussions about CF, still a relatively new disease; since then, dramatic

---

[7] Young had earlier studied renal physiology with Robert McCance, as previously noted.
[8] Corner's interest in ACTH treatment to prevent ROP helped push Silverman and Day to the first RCT in pediatrics, as previously noted.

Fig. 20.3 Dorothy
Andersen in 1956 at
Winifred Young's house in
Epsom, England.
(Courtesy of Archives &
Special Collections, Health
Sciences Library,
Columbia University)

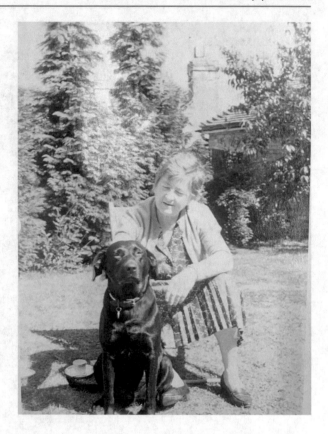

changes in European healthcare had occurred, as well as significant advances in medical knowledge generally. By 1956, CF clinical care and research was growing rapidly in Great Britain as well as in the rest of Europe, and her contributions were more broadly recognized.

It is worth remembering about Andersen that any contentment or satisfaction she enjoyed was always linked in some way to her social conscience, to her interest in leading a life which had meaning and benefit to others, a desire she shared with her parents.[9] However, her parents' lives were cut short by disease, and their aspirations may have been partly unfulfilled. Satisfaction for Andersen was not dependent on career advancement, or on leadership roles, or on organized religion: she wasn't frustrated by her slow advancement to the rank of University Professor, she had no leadership dreams beyond setting the research agenda in her own lab, and like her father, a strong ethical foundation overrode any spiritual concerns.

As a result, in the last decade of her life, Andersen must have felt some measure of satisfaction as she looked back, as she took some time to enjoy the view: no matter what else happened, she was proud of what she had accomplished for her patients

---

[9]Andersen mentioned in a Mount Holyoke College questionnaire in 1960 that one of the college attributes she most wanted to preserve was "a sense of public service."

and their families, she was equally proud of her work as a researcher, and she was content with a life lived by her own rules.

Or as content as any "Vermont farmer contemplating the amount of granite to be removed from a potential pasture" [10] could be.

References

1. Dorothy H. Andersen papers. Archives at the Augustus C. Long Health Sciences Library of Columbia University.
2. Machol L. Ahead of her time: a biography of Dorothy H. Andersen, M.D.
3. Presbyterian Hospital. Annual report of the Presbyterian Hospital in the City of New York. New York: The Presbyterian Hospital in the City of New York; 1939-64.
4. Ores C. Interview with Celia Ores, J.S. Baird, Editor. 2021.
5. Damrosch DS. Dorothy Hansine Andersen. J Pediatr. 1964;65:477–9.
6. Straus J, Strauss L. Rusty McIntosh by some of the many who experienced the essence of his presence at Babies Hospital, 1931–1960. Babies Hospital Alumni Association; 1987.
7. Katz M. Interview with Michael Katz., J.S. Baird, Editor. 2019.
8. Doershuk CF. Cystic fibrosis in the 20th century: people, events, and progress. Cleveland: AM Publishing Ltd; 2001.
9. Andersen DH. Lymphatics of the fallopian tube of the sow/by Dorothy H. Andersen, Contributions to embryology, vol. 19, no. 102. Washington, DC: Carnegie Institution of Washington; 1927.
10. Babies Hospital historical archives. Archives at the Augustus C. Long Health Sciences Library of Columbia University.

A Foundation and a Club for CF

21

In spite of a proliferation of CF research in the 1950s, untested or poorly tested therapies were still common. In large part, this was a consequence of the multisystem nature of the disease, as well as the rapid development of drug therapies in the twentieth century. Patients, their families, and their physicians were often left with many more questions than answers: what is the best way to utilize and/or deliver antibiotics, bronchodilators, and chest physiotherapy? What therapies are available for respiratory support? Do mist tents, steroids, or trypsin help with airway secretions or symptoms of lung disease? How should pancreatic enzymes and vitamins be dosed? These and many other questions – including the possibility of a disease cure – were central to the care of patients with CF, and answers were not easy to get.

As a result, parents and families began to band together, and regional organizations supporting CF care formed in the United States to help ensure the best clinical care for their children with CF and to keep families and the public informed about the disease. An early focus on education about CF, both for the public and for physicians, would eventually shift in the largest organizations to sponsored research into the disease.

In 1954, one regional organization in Philadelphia was poised to grow far beyond its boundaries; it included Dr. Milton Graub and his wife Evelyn (parents of a child with CF) and Dr. Wynne Sharples, "a local socialite and non-practicing pediatrician who was also the mother of two CF children" [1]. In 1955, Sharples helped obtain a charter to turn their regional organization into a national foundation, and a meeting was then held in Rustin McIntosh's office at Babies Hospital to determine the structure for this new foundation:

> Dr. Sharples immediately proposed that the Board of Trustees be made up of outstanding citizens whom she would designate… Dr. Sharples envisioned an elitist Board with the chapters raising the funds, but without representation. [1]

As this was unacceptable to several individuals in the meeting, a compromise was sought: "Dr. McIntosh and the legal counsel finally advised that equal

© The Author(s), under exclusive license to Springer Nature Switzerland AG 2022
J. S. Baird, *Dorothy Hansine Andersen*,
https://doi.org/10.1007/978-3-030-87484-1_21

representation seemed fair" [1]. The new organization was named the National CF Research Foundation (NCFRF) and incorporated as a not-for-profit health agency in Delaware [2], with 50% of the Board of Trustees made up of chapter representatives.

Sharples was chosen as its first President. Paul di Sant'Agnese described Sharples' value as NCFRF President:

> Dr. Sharples was very well connected socially and politically and succeeded in getting some of the powerful members of Congress interested in the problem. This eventually resulted in my recruitment in 1960 by the National Institutes of Health. [1]

Among Sharples' connections, George de Mohrenschildt – her husband at that time and the father of her two children – was a friend of the Bouvier family, including Jacqueline (Bouvier) Kennedy, Senator John F. Kennedy's wife.[1] Both the Bouvier family and de Mohrenschildt had extensive connections with European royalty, as did di Sant'Agnese; though such connections may have benefitted di Sant'Agnese, it is unclear if or how they benefitted this new foundation. It is also unclear why Andersen was not included in these initial negotiations.

In any case, Andersen joined the NCFRF at its inception in July 1955 as a member of the Medical Education Committee, which included Harry Shwachman, Paul di Sant'Agnese, and Paul Patterson. However di Sant'Agnese suggested that Andersen was not in favor of organizations like the NCFRF (Fig. 21.1):

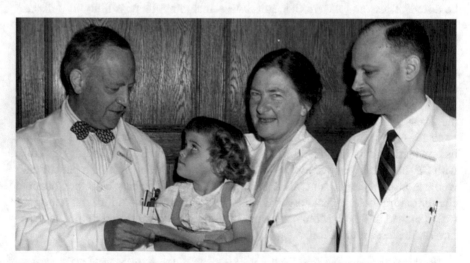

Fig. 21.1 Rustin McIntosh, Dorothy Andersen, and Paul di Sant'Agnese with a young patient. (Courtesy of Archives & Special Collections, Health Sciences Library, Columbia University)

---

[1] Interestingly, de Mohrenschildt was also a friend of Lee Harvey Oswald from 1962 through 1963, though he denied any role in John Kennedy's assassination during his extensive testimony before the Warren Commission.

Dr. Dorothy Andersen was against such an effort on our part as perhaps she felt physicians should not be involved in matters that did not directly concern the care of patients. Both Dr. Rustin McIntosh, the Chairman of Pediatrics at Babies Hospital and I tried many times to convince her, but she steadfastly refused to participate directly in any group activities. [1]

In spite of these comments (and in the absence of any evidence that McIntosh agreed with di Sant'Agnese's assessment), Andersen did participate extensively in NCFRF meetings and via correspondence, providing thoughtful answers to innumerable questions including routine requests to review handouts, scripts for publicity films, finished publicity films, foundation grants, and clinical guidelines.

Selections from Andersen's correspondence with Sharples are particularly revealing of Andersen's role within the NCFRF during its first few years [3]:

- *August 1956*: in response to Sharples offering "medical advice by mail" in June 1955 to a parent of a child with CF, Andersen wrote to Sharples reminding her that medical advice to a patient one has never examined and who is a patient of another physician "is sometimes counted as malpractice."
- *July 1958*: Sharples reprimanded Andersen: "It has just come to my attention that there is to be a symposium on cystic fibrosis at the pediatric meetings in Chicago this October. As a recipient of support from this Foundation, I would appreciate the National Foundation's being informed of the symposium and your participation in the program… A great deal of the present interest in cystic fibrosis is due to the work of the National Foundation and its chapters, and a large portion of the research being undertaken at present is supported by this organization. I would appreciate being informed of important medical events in connection with cystic fibrosis and the work of the Foundation."
- *August 1958*: Andersen responded to Sharples: "The reprimand in your letter of July 31st is based on a misapprehension. I have not for some years asked for or received a grant from the National Cystic Fibrosis Foundation. Academic freedom and freedom of expression are both dear to me. I appreciate your sincerity and the great effort which you have put into the Foundation. However, as your letter demonstrates, the Foundation has a rather imperious viewpoint. To avoid conflict I have sought and obtained funds for research from other sources. If you feel that it would make for greater harmony I shall be happy to resign from the Medical Education Committee."
- *September 1959*: Andersen was asked several times by Sharples to provide an opinion on the use of corticosteroid therapy in CF, as Sharples had heard about two children "with remarkable responses from steroid therapy." Andersen responded (gently) that such a question required careful clinical study before rendering an opinion. She noted "I should imagine that in some cases with highly resistant bacteria the use of cortisone would hasten a downhill course."
- *November 1959*: Andersen resigned from the Medical Education Committee, suggesting "the committee's function is poorly defined" and that there was a disconnect between the publicity and research aspects of the Foundation's mission: "We who are willing to spend some years to verify a point before

publication, lest we make a misstatement, are perhaps better off if we admire the techniques of publicity from afar."

- *December 1959*: Andersen was notified that Sharples had resigned as President.
- *January 1960*: Andersen requested an application form for a NCFRF research grant.
- *February 1960*: After being reassured by the new NCFRF President that Andersen's input was "highly valued," she accepted an invitation to rejoin the Medical Education Committee.

Reading between the lines, it appears that Andersen's concerns were generally consistent with the concerns of other responsible members of the NCFRF: Andersen became convinced that close collaboration with NCFRF attempts to publicize therapies not yet validated might cause more harm than good to patients, leading her to resign her Committee position. That was apparently a strong signal, and the foundation's President (Sharples) was quickly replaced. Andersen made no overt attempt to impose her will or to alter the NCFRF's mission; her insights into the relative roles of research and publicity were quite rational, and not motivated by a personal sense of vengeance or retribution.

Andersen's candor and honesty with Sharples is disarming and suggests the relationship between a mentor and a student, and not one between a researcher and a foundation president. Based solely on her correspondence with Andersen, Sharples may not have been well suited to her position at the NCFRF, but it is worth noting in her defense that she divorced de Mohrenschildt and then remarried early during her term as the foundation's President and that within a few months after she resigned as President, one of her two children with CF died [4]. Sharples' influence on the early course of the NCFRF has been described in positive terms, and she has been credited with being an effective fund-raiser [5], while Andersen's influence has been mostly unrecognized.

In 1978, a publication from the NIH referred to the early history of the NCFRF:

> From the beginning, the Foundation was blessed with two outstanding resources. One was a dedicated, involved and deeply committed Board of Trustees made up of parents and volunteers. The other major resource was the physicians who advised, directed, and formulated medical policies. Three of those who have been honored for their input and have been recognized as original medical founders are Dr. Harry Schwachman, Dr. Paul di Sant'Agnese and Dr. Paul Patterson. [6]

There was no mention of Dorothy Andersen by the NIH: only the men were honored. This was shabby treatment of the woman who authored the landmark 1938 study which defined the disease, who authored the studies designated here as her "CF firsts," as well as the 1951 and 1953 landmark studies leading to a new CF paradigm, and whose influence on the early direction taken by the foundation's leadership was mostly ignored. Andersen's omission was more than mere oversight and likely represents another expression of gender bias.

In 1959, Andersen decided to gather together a small group of physicians active in CF care and research, with the goal of better understanding the current state of the art in CF and discussing ongoing or future investigations in an informal atmosphere. Perhaps this was to some degree a response to Andersen's interactions with Sharples: instead of letting others set the CF research agenda, Andersen believed that CF clinicians and researchers should have an important role in that process. Perhaps it also reflected her recent experience with RCTs at Babies Hospital: Andersen knew that even the best academic physicians might be slow to accept the need for better evidence regarding untested therapies (e.g., corticosteroids in ROP or in CF). In any case, the first meeting at Buck Hill Falls in Pennsylvania included Andersen and Giulio Barbero, Paul di Sant'Agnese, LeRoy Matthews, Paul Patterson, and Harry Schwachman, among others. They decided to name this group the CF Club (which sounds like something Andersen would have promoted); it was a success according to di Sant'Agnese – and it continued to meet annually for several decades [1].

The judgment by di Sant'Agnese that Andersen refused to participate in CF organizations seems overly harsh and inconsistent with her role in the NCFRF, the CF club, as well as many other research and educational meetings, or her relationships with patients and their families. It is likely that Andersen in 1955 had the foresight to recognize potential difficulties associated with the new CF foundation (e.g., the conflict which emerged with Sharples) and that this insight was lost on di Sant'Agnese, perhaps even on McIntosh. In any case, any history of the NCFRF which neglects to honor Andersen for her contributions is, at best, inadequate.

As usual, whatever complaints were made about Andersen – including her participation or lack of participation with various groups – didn't seem to bother her. As the 1950s ended and a new decade began, her concerns were more fundamental: the end of an era at Babies Hospital and a rapid decline in her own health. She was, as a result, in even more haste to finish the work she had started.

References

1. Doershuk CF. Cystic fibrosis in the 20th century: people, events, and progress. Cleveland: AM Publishing Ltd; 2001.
2. Tulcin DF. Memoirs of a monarch. New York: iUniverse, Inc; 2008.
3. Dorothy H. Andersen papers. Archives at the Augustus C. Long Health Sciences Library of Columbia University.
4. George de Mohrenschildt. 2020 [cited 2020 October 15]. Available from: https://en.wikipedia.org/w/index.php?title=George_de_Mohrenschildt&oldid=977393514.
5. Trivedi BP. Breath from salt: a deadly genetic disease, a new era in science, and the patients and families who changed medicine forever. BenBella Books, Incorporated; 2020.
6. National Institutes of Health. Cystic fibrosis: state of the art and directions for future research efforts. Department of Health, Education, and Welfare, Public Health Service, National Institutes of Health; 1978.

The End of an Era

22

Rustin McIntosh retired on June 30, 1960, at 65 years of age from Babies Hospital and Columbia University and soon moved his family out to their country home in the Berkshires: farming, winemaking, hiking, camping – these rural pleasures and more, along with chamber music, writing and editing, and travel, as well as a massive correspondence, would all add to his responsibilities during retirement. This time, there was no reconsideration, no negotiation which would bring him back: the McIntosh Era at Babies Hospital was truly over.

Though his retirement was expected, most of the Babies Hospital faculty did not view the prospect dispassionately: tributes and reminiscences to McIntosh were written by many of them. Each of these tributes bears testament to the good will and the fervent devotion they shared regarding the McIntosh Era: William Silverman's essay "In search of the spirit of Babies Hospital" [1], Douglas Damrosch's essay "Highlight- Rustin McIntosh" [2], and a commemorative volume "The McIntosh Era at Babies Hospital, 1931–1960" [3] all appeared around the time he retired, while memorials following his death in 1986 included Douglas Damrosch's essay "A tribute to Rustin McIntosh, M.D. [4]" and a collection of reminiscences: "Rusty McIntosh by some of the many who experienced the essence of his presence at Babies Hospital, 1931–1960" [5]. The admiration and longing manifest in these tributes help explain another response: several faculty members left or retired from Columbia University and Babies Hospital within a year of McIntosh's retirement, including Virginia Apgar, John Caffey, Paul di Sant'Agnese, Charles May, and Conrad Riley.

After 30 years at the helm of both Columbia University's Department of Pediatrics and Babies Hospital, McIntosh had put his stamp on both (somewhat similar to Holt's legacy, as remembered by McIntosh: "Dr. Holt for many years was Babies Hospital"). As Douglas Damrosch wrote: "Babies Hospital is Rusty's hospital and its standards of patient care, pediatric teaching, and scientific investigation are his standards or as close to them as those privileged to serve under him have been able to achieve" [2]. Babies Hospital during the McIntosh Era was arguably

© The Author(s), under exclusive license to Springer Nature Switzerland AG 2022
J. S. Baird, *Dorothy Hansine Andersen*,
https://doi.org/10.1007/978-3-030-87484-1_22

one of the most important children's hospitals in the United States, and McIntosh was its leader.

With his conservative nature, it is ironic that much of McIntosh's leadership success, as perceived by others, appeared to derive from his support for a free-thinking approach to the acquisition of knowledge. William Silverman was interviewed years later and said: "Rusty McIntosh certainly played a very big role in my life... The one thing I've said over and over is not one of these people [at Babies Hospital] that I admire so was a team player. None of them were team players. They were individualists, you know, and I think that probably explains my life-long problem with team-think" [6]. Damrosch wrote something similar: "As for me: Rusty was the most important man in my life. Very early in my house staff years I realized that I was attempting to emulate Rusty, knowing that I must fall short of the mark" [4], and also: "In such an atmosphere of healthy skepticism [at Babies Hospital], where 'authority' was never accepted for its own sake, research efforts had to be forward moving, rather than simply confirmations of the obvious" [4].

McIntosh's essentially parental attitude toward Babies Hospital was in large part responsible for his strong defense of Andersen and pediatric pathology during the crisis of 1949: he did not act selfishly – or at least wholly selfishly – in that conflict. Rather he perceived great value in keeping her at Babies Hospital where her talents, connections, and skills were converted into actual benefit to patients and ultimately to the practice of medicine generally; indeed, McIntosh began to refer to Andersen in the 1940s as a member of the Department of Pediatrics (though her primary appointment was still in the Department of Pathology). McIntosh was well aware how Andersen had changed the way medicine was practiced in twentieth-century United States. If McIntosh had not succeeded in that 1949 crisis regarding Andersen and lab space, it is possible that the CF sweat studies might have been delayed, at the very least. Conversely, though no evidence exists to suggest that Andersen shared greatly in the deep sadness and regret felt by many of her colleagues at McIntosh's retirement, she certainly recognized the value of his leadership and his support for her career. Fortunately, she was able to continue her research without a pause following his retirement; she was, by the 1960s, a full Professor at Columbia University with several research sponsors, and was as a result always able to set her own research agenda.

Neither McIntosh nor Andersen required reassurance about their conduct or interests or the perception by others of their academic import: neither one suffered from a lack of self-confidence (though Andersen was generally self-deprecatory in public). They were both unlikely to leave behind any evidence of their relationship – or lack of one – as neither had a habit of pointing out another's defects or needlessly extolling another's virtues. Theirs was a somewhat distant relationship built on respect and mutual recognition of the value each had in the world of academic medicine. Neither felt the need to further define this relationship. Perhaps if Andersen had survived into retirement, things might have been different; but that did not happen. It is intriguing that McIntosh, who survived Andersen by more than two decades, never offered more insight into his relationship with her.

In any case, Babies Hospital benefitted from McIntosh's subtle diplomatic skills:

In fact, his [McIntosh's] skill in diplomacy eventually became legendary, as did the personal attributes which diplomacy requires and which he had in abundance: integrity, quiet geniality, forthright manner, ability to put down inept reasoning with logic and to keep argument to the point. [4]

These defensive and diplomatic skills were not McIntosh's only leadership skills. William Bauman described another special ability:

His [McIntosh's] ability to capitalize on rivalries among his staff- particularly the distaff-leading each to out-perform the other and bring fame and glory to themselves and to Babies Hospital... particularly the ladies of H. influenza and Cystic Fibrosis. [5]

The suggestion that McIntosh might have subtly encouraged Hattie Alexander and Dorothy Andersen to compete with each other warrants some comment.

Michael Katz, who knew both women, was mentored by Alexander and invited by Andersen to visit her farm, and later served as Chair of Pediatrics at Columbia University, was definitive that they did not compete in public and were only ever gracious and respectful toward each other [7]. It is possible that Bauman's and Katz's observations were both correct and that these talented women were careful not to admit competitive influences, at least in public. There is no firm evidence available to support the notion that McIntosh capitalized "on rivalries among his staff," including, in particular, women.

Nevertheless, any exploration of the place of women in academic pediatrics during the McIntosh Era at Babies Hospital requires some knowledge of McIntosh's attitudes toward women. William Silverman said in an interview that "many people have said to me that Rusty McIntosh didn't hire many women" [6], though he added: "But many stars in the department were women." Is it possible that gender bias characterized some of McIntosh's interactions with the Babies Hospital faculty?

Several reasons to doubt gender bias on McIntosh's part exist:

• A renowned faculty member, Melvin Grumbach, remembered:

Rusty was way ahead of his time in terms of supporting women [in medicine]. He already had women that he mentored on his faculty and fostered their advancement... They all went up the ladder. That was way back, and that was a period when as you know, there were few women in medicine... I think [his wife] Millicent had an effect on his view about women in the profession. [8]

McIntosh's wife Millicent was the Dean and eventually President of Barnard College at Columbia University and was described in *The New York Times* in 1998 as "a feminist role model for women in the 1940's and 50's who wanted to combine family and career" [9]. McIntosh was supportive of the careers of the women physicians he supervised at Babies Hospital, as he was supportive of his wife's career.

• In 1974, Bauman suggested to Elizabeth Ufford (then president of the Alumni Association at Babies Hospital and long-time companion of Hattie Alexander) that "The Babies Hospital has been outstanding in its hospitality to aspiring women pediatricians long before women's lib was heard of, and that during that time some 'giants' among women pediatricians were trained and encouraged" [10]. Ufford began planning a speech on outstanding women physicians at Babies Hospital and asked for McIntosh's opinion. His response was illuminating, as he discussed and praised not just Andersen and Alexander, Wollstein and Beryl Paige, but also Helen Ranney, Katherine Dodge Brownell, and other women who trained or worked at Babies Hospital prior to a successful academic career. He recalled Dorothy Reed's service as a resident at Babies Hospital and suggested that she was "the first one [of the Babies Hospital residents] you should mention."[1] McIntosh was cognizant and supportive of several different generations of women physicians who had been associated with Babies Hospital.

- McIntosh published generous tributes to both Wollstein [11] and Alexander [12] after their deaths. He corresponded frequently with Hilde Bruch [10] and enjoyed playing chamber music with Virginia Apgar during his retirement (he described her as "a violist whose boundless enthusiasm bridged whatever gap might lie in her technical competence" [13]). It is true that his relationship with Andersen was not as easy to characterize. However, he remained supportive of the legacies of the women physicians he had supervised at Babies Hospital throughout his professional life, and many of them had successful careers in academic medicine beyond Columbia University.
- McIntosh authored a short book in 1980 which offered a glowing account of Helen Rich [13]: a vibrant, nurturing, champion of classical chamber music (at whose soirees both McIntosh and his family, as well as Virginia Apgar, were participants). McIntosh's non-academic interests appeared to be immune to some of the common gender biases of his era.
- Lastly, Babies Hospital was founded and originally run by women physicians, and some of the motivation and energy they shared in its establishment likely persisted as a kind of institutional heritage. McIntosh knew and respected that heritage.

In the final analysis, gender bias was a common social problem during the decades of the McIntosh Era, and Andersen's legacy seems to reflect this problem. Though it is not easy to ascertain the presence of gender bias at Babies Hospital, it is likely that McIntosh's influence was not always benign. How much he was able to help move the balance of this problem toward a greater participation by women in academic medicine is unclear, though it is reasonable to grant him some progress overall.

Even in retirement, McIntosh continued to have significant demands placed on his time. As Damrosch wrote:

Rusty has retired but in fact this could not be further from the truth; we hear that he is as busy as ever, dividing his time between the latest edition of Holt and McIntosh and his office as Special Consultant to the New York City Department of Health. [2]

---

[1] McIntosh may have been unaware then that Wollstein was the first resident physician at Babies Hospital.

The repercussions of his retirement reverberated for years through Babies Hospital, as well as through the world of academic pediatrics generally: no one wanted to see him leave the public stage, and this meant that he received numerous requests to speak, to moderate, to visit, and to advise. He was eventually forced to limit his responses to many of these requests due to the large demand and in order to continue to enjoy some part of his retirement. It was hard for him to limit his correspondence: he wrote back to just about anyone who solicited his help, and that seemed to include just about anyone in academic pediatrics.

Edward Curnen was recruited from the University of North Carolina (where he had been the first Chair of Pediatrics) to replace McIntosh, and he joined Babies Hospital as Carpentier Professor of Pediatrics and Chair of Pediatrics at Columbia University's College of Physicians and Surgeons in 1960. Curnen was a researcher in infectious diseases, particularly viruses, and had been an assistant at the Rockefeller Institute (where he also worked with Oswald Avery and Colin MacLeod). He was one of the first to recognize the importance of Coxsackie virus in the production of human disease. He was a friend of Hattie Alexander before coming to Babies Hospital and shared several of her research interests. Babies Hospital faculty continued to be productive in both medical research and education during his tenure.

But the McIntosh Era at Babies Hospital was truly over.

References

1. Silverman WA. In search of the spirit of Babies Hospital. In: Babies Hospital, editor. Babies Hospital historical collection, 1887–1994. Archives at the Augustus C. Long Health Sciences Library of Columbia University.
2. Damrosch DS. Highlight-Rustin McIntosh. Alumni Association Bulletin, College of Physicians and Surgeons, Columbia University; 1961. VI.
3. McIntosh R. The McIntosh era at Babies Hospital, 1931–1960: a commemorative volume to honor Rustin McIntosh. Babies Hospital; 1960.
4. Damrosch DS. A tribute to Rustin McIntosh, M.D., C.-P.M. Center, Editor. 1986.
5. Straus J, Strauss L. Rusty McIntosh by some of the many who experienced the essence of his presence at Babies Hospital, 1931–1960. Babies Hospital Alumni Association; 1987.
6. Silverman WA. Oral history project: William A. Sliverman, MD, L.M. Gartner, Editor. American Academy of Pediatrics; 1997.
7. Katz M. Interview with Michael Katz., J.S. Baird, Editor. 2019.
8. Grumbach MM. Oral history project: Melvin M. Grumbach, M.B. Abbott, Editor. American Academy of Pediatrics; 2013.
9. Arenson KW. Feminist's Centennial. In: The New York Times. New York; 1998.
10. Rustin McIntosh papers. Archives at the Augustus C. Long Health Sciences Library of Columbia University.
11. M. R. Martha Wollstein, M.D. 1868-1939. Am J Dis Child. 1939;58(6):1301–1.
12. McIntosh R. Hattie Alexander. Pediatrics. 1968;42(3):544.
13. McIntosh R. Helen rice: the great lady of chamber music. Burlington: Amateur Chamber Music Players/George Little; 1980.

Though she was open, honest, and friendly with most people she met, Dorothy Andersen was also a private person: without any close family, single and childless, and devoted to her work, she did not easily share the details of her private life – except with a few close friends. She left hardly any records of her non-academic life, preferring instead to let her work speak for her. So when she first recognized that something was seriously wrong with her health, and when she was first seen and then diagnosed with lung cancer, and what her treatment included – none of that information is available.

Smoking in the United States was much more widespread in the 1950s than in any previous decade, in part as cigarettes were by then mass produced and in association with changes in social custom. Smoking for women conferred some sense of independence, of flouting older traditions; Andersen was a smoker, and not in moderation during the decade prior to her death. The evidence of an association between smoking and lung cancer or heart disease became progressively more convincing in the 1950s, culminating in 1964 – the year after Andersen's death – in the US Surgeon General's report documenting the health hazards of smoking in a way that soon changed attitudes: declines in smoking over several years eventually were associated with declines in lung cancer rates. Though Andersen was certainly aware of the emerging data linking smoking with lung cancer (almost all of this data involved studies in men), by the time the dangers of smoking were clear to her, it was too late.

Celia Ores remembered about Andersen's smoking in 1960 that "she only needed one light in the morning" [1], implying that she chain-smoked most of the day. She also recalled one of Andersen's afternoon tea meetings[1] in which research projects were reviewed: when the discussion turned to new topics, Sidney Blumenthal suggested "Why don't we talk about Dr. Andersen's smoking?" Andersen answered: "I'm very fond of you Sidney, but if you are going to behave like this I can't have you back to my tea" [1].

---

[1] It is likely that the focus for these meetings was Andersen's research agenda in pediatric cardiology and that it occurred sometime between 1960 and 1962.

It was likely sometime in 1961 [2] at around 60 years of age (though it may have been a few months later in 1962 [3]) that Andersen underwent surgery, with a biopsy of her lungs: she was diagnosed with cancer. Ores recalled that she later met the surgeon who operated on Andersen and that this surgery occurred perhaps a year prior to Andersen's death: the surgeon was, Ores recalled, a Hopkins graduate and a classmate of Andersen's, and "when he opened her chest, the disease was everywhere" [1]. He realized "there was nothing he could do to help her" and quickly finished the surgery [1].

Though no information about Andersen's actual diagnosis is available, lung cancer associated with smoking is usually of the non-small cell type; most do not respond well to chemotherapy or radiation therapy (though this was not known in the early 1960s), and long-term survival was poor: most patients then survived for less than a year. Surgical resection of the tumor was the primary therapy available, and according to Ores' account, that did not happen due to extensive disease.

By 1961, Andersen began to receive invitations to dinners and meetings to honor her medical contributions. It would not be at all surprising if some knowledge of her illness had leaked out, inspiring some recognition of her value to the academic medicine community. An interesting photo in October 1961 shows her at a dinner in her honor given by the Department of Pathology at Columbia University: a sea of mostly elderly, dour men in tuxedos surrounds her. Her expression is somewhat amused yet firm, an interesting contrast to her earlier image as the "Brew mistress" with glug and a cigarette (Fig. 23.1).

Shortly after being diagnosed with lung cancer, she quit smoking. As a result, Andersen told Hilde Bruch that "the sweets and chewing gum she substituted for cigarettes were affecting her teeth and gums, and that she was probably the only cancer patient who gained rather than lost weight" [2].

While much of 1962 was taken up with the preparation of manuscripts for publication, she continued to spend time at her farm: it was likely late that summer that she reshingled the roof of the main house with Peg Miller (Marion Beman Chute's daughter, then a junior in college; Miller noted that Andersen also taught her how to cook on the wood stove during the same visit [4]). A month later, in September 1962, Andersen and Hilde Bruch enjoyed a dinner at Andersen's farm of stuffed Cornish game hens [3] cooked on the wood stove. On her return home, Andersen asked Bruch to examine (feel or palpate) her liver, as Andersen thought it felt "bumpy" [2]: Bruch refused, and Andersen then saw a physician who suggested a biopsy. Andersen refused the biopsy, knowing the implications of this new finding: it strongly suggested that the cancer had metastasized to her liver and that suggested to her that she did not have long to live. She discussed the likelihood of her imminent death with her close friends and suggested it was unfortunate because she still had much work to do and hoped to be able to enjoy more of her life at this age [2]. Such conversations with close friends occurred mostly at the farm, where Andersen "kept beers cooling outside on the window sill to enjoy beer sessions and poker games" [3].

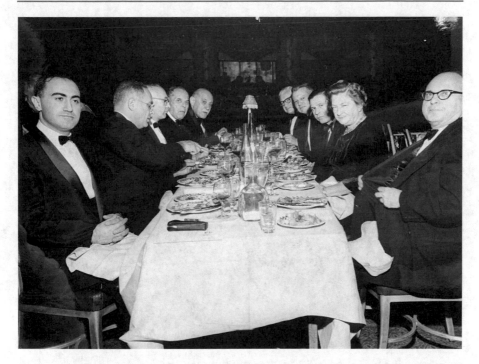

Fig. 23.1 Faculty from Columbia University's Department of Pathology at a dinner for Dorothy Andersen (seated second from right) in the Waldorf-Astoria hotel in New York City, October 1961. (Courtesy of Archives & Special Collections, Health Sciences Library, Columbia University)

Based on rather thin evidence, it has been suggested that Andersen "after hours, drank hard" [5], with an implication that alcohol played a large part in her life. After all, she was a chain-smoker, whose friends drank beers (or occasionally something even stronger [6]) with her at the farm, and she was well-known for her winter glug parties at Babies Hospital. This seems to be another instance in which Andersen's behavior was judged by someone else's standards. She lived her life as she wanted, and she did not care to modify her behavior in order to please others. There is no evidence that alcohol was a problem for her, and all indications suggest that she used it mainly in social situations, perhaps to help relieve stress[2].

In January 1963 Andersen went to Philadelphia to accept the Great Heart Award from the Variety Club of Philadelphia for her "humanitarian work with children" [7]; the singer Patti Page also received an award. By then Andersen had lost weight and she appears frail and a bit thin, even in comparison to Page (Fig. 23.2).

The cancer was by then advancing rapidly: for over a month, she had been having difficulty walking or doing even the simplest tasks. On returning home "she was unable to carry her suitcase upstairs" [3]. She was briefly hospitalized, suggesting

[2] Celia Ores affirmed in an interview that she never saw Andersen drunk and that Andersen did not have a problem with alcohol.

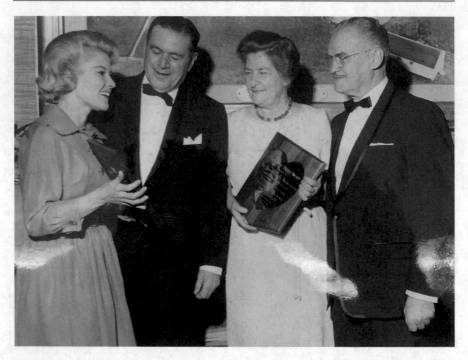

Fig. 23.2 Patti Page and Dorothy Andersen being honored in Philadelphia by the Variety Club in January 1963. (Courtesy of Archives & Special Collections, Health Sciences Library, Columbia University)

to others that it was for a circulatory disorder, and refused to use a wheelchair. It is likely she made several brief visits to her lab/office at Babies Hospital when few of her colleagues were around; she may even have taken the opportunity to type out a few pages about her life and work.

Early in 1963 Mount Holyoke College received a short autobiographical sketch "by Andy" [8]; it is possible that she [7] completed this in response to a specific request from a friend who knew the extent of her illness, though the sketch was undated and at least some of it had been written several years earlier. As was her practice, this sketch was written in the third person using a humorous and self-deprecating style. Barely two pages in length, she only hinted at her extensive work outside the realm of CF: "Dr. Andersen finds the wealth of unexplored problems in pediatric pathology rather distracting and occasionally interrupts the pursuit of the celiac syndrome to study and report interesting cases" [8]. There was no acknowledgment of her illness, and the second page ended with a brief paragraph about her farm, with the last sentence seeming to suggest that more was to follow: "It is also a fine place for birds, photography, sketching, cooking, eating, and conversation" [8].

By February her health began to deteriorate even more rapidly, "as her appetite and weight loss announced the seriousness of her condition" [3]. It is easy to envision her declining at home while reassuring friends that all was well: therapeutic options were much more limited for the treatment of cancer in the 1960s. She was stoic, and not given to complaints: as the end of her life drew near, her chief concern was not to bother or distract others. As noted by Douglas Damrosch: "She conducted her campaign against this illness with the same rugged spirit with which she had tackled earlier problems. Characteristically, she shouldered the full burden herself" [9]. She was admitted to Presbyterian Hospital and likely told very few. Bruch was away at a meeting in Baltimore. Ores remembered that Andersen called her on the phone from her hospital bed the night before her death in order to discuss Ores' future career.

Andersen's hospitalization was brief: she passed away there on March 3, 1963. She was only 61 years old. Her colleagues and friends were stunned and grief-stricken, including those few who knew she was ill. Andersen's absence affected them all deeply: some, like Ores[3], lost an academic mentor as well as a friend, while others, like Bruch[4], lost a friend and a guide who offered valuable counsel and served as a role model. Sidney Blumenthal[5] realized that he had lost an important collaborator in the development of pediatric cardiology, while Carolyn Denning's[6] loss of her research mentor was overshadowed by her growing awareness of some of the difficulties inherent in managing an extensive CF practice at a large academic medical center. Friends outside of Andersen's professional circle mourned the loss of someone always loyal and thoughtful and ready to help, whose interests and skills were anything but common.

Though there was no sense of loneliness in Andersen's life, the few facts available regarding her death suggest a different story at the end: Andersen's private and stoic nature coupled with her concern to avoid causing others distress appear to have led her to endure the pain and suffering of her last few days and weeks mostly alone. Andersen was buried at Oak Woods Cemetery in Chicago (where her parents, maternal grandparents, and maternal great grandparents are also buried).

Andy's abandoned farm was left to Marion Beman Chute, whose family continued to enjoy it for decades. In 1968, Chute sold a large portion of the original

---

[3] Ores' subsequent medical career was focused mostly on CF, and she remained affiliated with Columbia University's Department of Pediatrics.

[4] Within a year of Andersen's death, Bruch left Columbia University after purchasing a slightly used 1959 Silver Cloud Rolls Royce: her nephew Herbert drove her in the Rolls all the way to Texas (by way of New Orleans) where she accepted the post of Professor of Psychiatry at Baylor University's College of Medicine. She eventually authored several books on eating disorders which contributed significantly to her academic legacy. The somewhat freewheeling nature of Bruch's lifestyle after Andersen's death seemed to owe something to Andersen's influence.

[5] Blumenthal left Babies Hospital for the University of Miami School of Medicine in the early 1970s, where he was later named Dean of Continuing Education. In 1976 he left Miami to accept the position of Director of the Heart and Vascular Disease Division of the National Heart, Lung, and Blood Institute at the National Institutes of Health.

[6] Denning later served as the Director of Babies Hospital's Cystic Fibrosis and Pediatric Pulmonary Disease Center before transferring many of the clinic patients and staff from Babies Hospital to St. Vincent's Hospital in New York City in 1977.

acreage to help defray the tax burden [4]. Chute's daughter Margaret (Peg) Miller donated the remainder to the New Jersey Natural Lands Trust in 2013 and that now forms a part of the Reinhardt Preserve adjacent to High Point State Park. Many of Andersen's remaining assets were distributed among her friends and colleagues. Bess Haskell was the executrix of Andersen's estate, and she helped direct some of the posthumous income from publishing back to Columbia University [10].

A tribute to Andersen's career by her colleague Douglas Damrosch appeared in the Journal of Pediatrics [9]. Though McIntosh offered tributes to Martha Wollstein and Hattie Alexander following their deaths, he seemed hesitant to say much after Andersen's death. Perhaps he believed that his 1949 resignation in defense of Andersen was sufficient evidence of his respect and concern; or perhaps grief prevented him from making any published response. Houston Merritt, then Dean of Columbia University's medical school, offered the following: "All of us mourn the passing of our colleague and I especially, since I have known Dorothy since she was a classmate of mine at Johns Hopkins" [8]. Within a week of her death, the faculty of Columbia University's College of Physicians and Surgeons adopted a resolution recording "its deep sense of loss in the death of Dr. Andersen and its deep sympathy for her friends in their bereavement" [10]. The responses from CF families expressed a deeper truth: "We have lost a wonderful friend in Dr. Andersen" [8].

In April 1963, 1 month after Andersen's death, Babies Hospital celebrated its 75th anniversary. There was an elaborate dinner at the Waldorf Astoria Hotel in New York City, and Distinguished Service Medals were awarded to Hattie Alexander, Dorothy Andersen, John Caffey, Richard Day, Rustin McIntosh, and Ashley Weech (Fig. 23.3).

This event was freighted with the weight of multiple endings: Andersen's recent death, McIntosh's retirement several years earlier, as well as the fact that only one of the honorees was still working at Babies Hospital (Alexander), and her career was drawing to a close. In his memorial comments at the dinner, Douglas Damrosch noted about Andersen:

> She carried a service and teaching load which would have bowed less sturdy shoulders and the only complaints heard from her were the sort of dry, laconic remarks that you would expect from a Vermont farmer contemplating the amount of granite to be removed from a potential pasture. [10]

Some of the qualities commonly attributed to Andersen include those attributes frequently ascribed to Vermont farmers: she was stoic, laconic, and a hard worker who did not complain. However, the qualities identified in her father, including loyalty, candor, and honesty as well as a self-effacing nature, seem to better characterize much of her professional life. One of her friends (Bess Haskell) later suggested that "She was such a versatile, brilliant but unassuming person" [8]: self-effacing, unassuming, and even self-deprecatory – any of these might be used to describe her demeanor.

It is worth remembering about Andersen that the loss of both her parents while still a teenager did not lead her to despair, but rather to a better appreciation of the

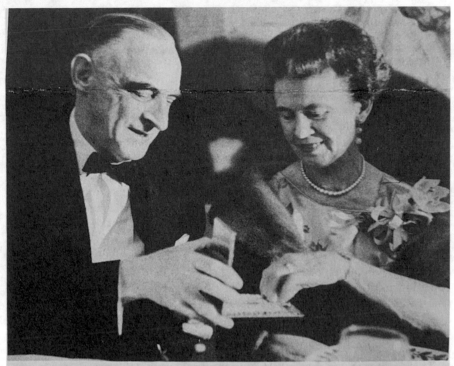

General Lucius D. Clay offers a cigarette to Dr. Hattie E. Alexander, who was awarded a Distinguished Service Medal.

Fig. 23.3 At the 75th anniversary of Babies Hospital in April, 1963. (Courtesy of Archives & Special Collections, Health Sciences Library, Columbia University)

fragile nature of life; she began to consider medicine as a career. An independent streak, manifest as a lack of concern about appearances, an interest in living life on her own terms, and her inability to always accept conventional wisdom contributed to her enjoyment of life in the face of adversity and to her concern about scientific truth, as well as to her interest in surgical training. Early training as an anatomist emphasized the value of work which is careful and thorough. As a result, Andersen's unique approach throughout her career included the meticulous and rigorous skills of an anatomist and pathologist, the sympathetic and thoughtful nature of a clinician, and the insightful and imaginative skills of a researcher.

Though medicine and science in the United States seemed to be joined at the hip in the twentieth century, reflecting in part the impact of the Johns Hopkins University medical school, the Rockefeller Institute, and the Flexner report, something like a divorce developed within just a few decades. Jules Hirsch, former physician-in-chief at the Rockefeller Institute's hospital, opined in 1997 about this "divorce of science and medicine":

those scientific advances most relevant to the amelioration of human disease may no longer be generated by clinicians, although clinicians will use products generated by the findings of laboratory scientists for the care of their patients. If this analysis is correct, then a long historical connection between attending to the sick and the development of biologic science will come to an end in our time. [11]

Andersen's career suggested the path that she used in reconciling "attending to the sick" with "the development of biologic science." Andersen's research as a pathologist led her to identify a new disease, and she then became a clinician caring for children with this disease; she subsequently undertook research needed to help advance medical knowledge and care for these sick children. However, this path required not just expertise in all the skills required in a lab and a clinic or hospital but also the ability to do productive research, including insights into pathophysiology, understanding the importance of hypothesis-driven investigations, and the resources to carry out these investigations.

Andersen's unusual skillset enabled her to be successful as a pathologist, a clinician, and a researcher and to handle any attendant concerns with relative ease (e.g., research funding, foreign languages, and conflicts with related organizations). This practitioner skillset is, however, uncommon – even in the world of academic medicine – and her path to success is not an easy one to follow. As our understanding and appreciation of biologic science increases over time, this path will be much harder to follow; it is even more difficult in the presence of any kind of bias against the practitioner.

The identification of gender bias on the part of historical persons no longer available to defend themselves is tricky: how strong is the evidence? It is possible that refusal to offer membership in the Rockefeller Institute to Martha Wollstein was an example of gender bias; it is even possible that Wollstein was not promoted to professor at Columbia University due to gender bias, though specific evidence is lacking. It is clear that the refusal to offer Andersen or Virginia Apgar further surgical training involved gender bias. Belittling or minimizing Andersen's clinical skills, calling her a "self-proclaimed expert," and omitting her from a list of honorees associated with the CF Foundation all suggest gender bias. In addition, minimizing Andersen's role in the studies which helped identify CF sweat abnormalities while crediting Paul di Sant'Agnese appears to be an example of the Matilda effect, a particularly dismaying form of gender bias.

By the end of the 1960s, many of the Babies Hospital faculty that achieved fame during the McIntosh Era had either moved on, retired, or died. In particular, many of the women who made up this renowned generation of researchers and practitioners – including Andersen's colleagues Hattie Alexander, Virginia Apgar, and Hilde Bruch – were gone. Each of these remarkable women physicians – as well as Martha Wollstein, Beryl Paige, and others – devoted most of their adult lives to their careers. Their academic heritage was recognized for some of them during their lifetimes, but their personal lives were often poorly documented; for Andersen, at least, few were left to offer praise, to defend her legacy, or to offer some insight into her life and work.

Memorials for some of these extraordinary women were established and include an annual lecture at Columbia University in honor of Hattie Alexander, an award for a medical school graduate at Baylor University in honor of Hilde Bruch, and an Academy of Medical Educators at Columbia University in honor of Virginia Apgar. The contributions of Martha Wollstein and Beryl Paige remain mostly unrecognized, and Dorothy Andersen seems to have dropped off the academic map entirely following her death, her many interests and accomplishments seemingly forgotten or ignored: some kind of memorial to her at Columbia University is long overdue. Even a portrait of her by Frank Slater (painted shortly after her death) has disappeared from the hospital walls.

It is tempting to ascribe some social upheaval, some external force contributing to the success of Andersen and her female colleagues. Perhaps some common set of circumstances pushed each to achieve at extraordinary levels: several of them had in common the schools they attended and the training they received. Babies Hospital during the McIntosh Era certainly provided a unique setting for the talents and skills of several of these physicians to emerge. However, the truth is simpler: women were always waiting for opportunities to participate and excel in academic medicine, and Andersen and her colleagues were able to take advantage of some of the advances made by previous generations of women physicians and extend them in an environment that was a bit more receptive.

Dorothy Andersen was a "world-class" physician, equally at home as a clinician, a researcher, and a teacher. Her lack of self-importance was not affected by her many accomplishments, and detractors never seemed to bother her. I believe her accomplishments deserve a wider stage and that her approach to life, including the intelligence, honesty, dedication, and bravery she brought to that task, was heroic.

And for most of her career, Dorothy Andersen was indeed the most knowledgeable physician about CF.

References

1. Ores C. Interview with Celia Ores, J.S. Baird, Editor. 2021.
2. Bruch JH. Unlocking the Golden cage: an intimate biography of Hilde Bruch, M.D. Gürze Books; 1996.
3. Sicherman B, Green CH. Notable American women: the modern period: a biographical dictionary. Cambridge, MA: The Belknap Press of Harvard University Press; 1980.
4. Miller MP. History of Andy's farm, M. Rapp, Editor. 2013.
5. Trivedi BP. Breath from salt: a deadly genetic disease, a new era in science, and the patients and families who changed medicine forever. BenBella Books, Incorporated; 2020.
6. Ores C. Reading Pushkin in Siberia. Lulu Publishing Services; 2016.
7. Yan D, Holt PR. Willem Dicke. Brilliant clinical observer and translational investigator. Discoverer of the toxic cause of celiac disease. Clin Transl Sci. 2009;2(6):446–8.
8. Dorothy H. Andersen papers. Archives at the Augustus C. Long Health Sciences Library of Columbia University.
9. Damrosch DS. Dorothy Hansine Andersen. J Pediatr. 1964;65:477–9.
10. Babies Hospital historical archives. Archives at the Augustus C. Long Health Sciences Library of Columbia University.
11. Hirsch J. The role of clinical investigation in medicine: historical perspective from the Rockefeller University. Perspect Biol Med. 1997;41:108–17.

Afterword

While working as a pediatric intensivist at St. Vincent's Hospital in New York City, I began to feel a debt of gratitude to Dorothy Andersen: I was frequently drawn back to her original studies as I tried to understand more about CF. I was privileged to meet several people from the CF Center at St. Vincent's who knew Andersen, including Carolyn Denning: she trained under Andersen at Babies Hospital and came with the CF Center when it moved from Babies Hospital to St. Vincent's Hospital in 1977. With the help of several of the physicians at the CF Center (Jack Jacoby, Patricia Walker, and Maria Berdella), I learned something about caring for CF patients and was thrilled to meet Paul Quinton at a CF Foundation annual meeting. The stories of many of the patients and staff at St. Vincent's CF Center deserve to be told in some detail, as they were inspirational to me- perhaps one day.

As I learned more about CF, it often seemed odd that there wasn't more recognition of Dorothy Andersen's role in the history of that disease. Any reference to her 1938 study often emphasized the important contributions of other investigators, while many of her studies from the 1940s which helped define the field of CF care (what I have chosen to call her "CF firsts") were rarely mentioned, and one of the key observations about CF – the occurrence of dehydration and hypochloremia in CF patients during a heat wave in New York City – was frequently attributed incorrectly to Paul di Sant'Agnese. Any involvement by her in the subsequent CF sweat studies of 1953 was minimized or ignored. As I began to collect material for this biography, I was dismayed to discover that several physicians even found her behavior difficult and arrogant but was relieved to find no significant evidence supporting this assessment.

As the CF Foundation's role in this biography was only peripheral to the story of Dorothy Andersen's life, I have neglected to mention some of their recent successes. The Foundation (known as the NCFRF in the 1950s) supported a variety of critically important research efforts, including the development of an enzyme to break down the DNA in viscous airway secretions of patients with CF, the discovery of the CFTR gene, and the amazing development of therapies designed to cure CF by working inside affected cells: these drugs which improve CFTR function were developed by pharmaceutical companies in partnership with the Foundation. The

J. S. Baird, *Dorothy Hansine Andersen*, https://doi.org/10.1007/978-3-030-87484-1

Foundation now serves as a model for other philanthropic organizations and continues to play an important role in CF care.

My own career in medicine would not have been possible without Andrew Frantz, who interviewed me for medical school; he was the son of Virginia Kneeland Frantz, the first woman accepted for a surgical internship at CUMC. As a medical student at Columbia, I felt intimidated by Michael Katz (then Chair of the Department of Pediatrics); however that was my fault, and not his. As one of only a few eyewitnesses to the McIntosh Era still around, his excellent memory and kind words helped me feel more comfortable trying to describe a time and place I could never see. He mentioned several times to me that both Dorothy H ansine Andersen and Hattie Alexander were "world-class" physicians and researchers and suggested that both deserved more recognition than they got. I agree wholeheartedly with this sentiment.

When I returned to CUMC later in my career, I began to slowly piece together the puzzle of Dorothy Hansine Andersen, Babies Hospital, and cystic fibrosis. It took me a while, but I hope that this biography serves to reignite interest in Andersen: "It is a matter worth considering, at any rate" [1].

Reference

1. Andersen DH. Lymphatics of the fallopian tube of the sow/by Dorothy H. Andersen, Contributions to embryology, vol. 19, no. 102. Washington, DC: Carnegie Institution of Washington; 1927.

Index

Printed in the United States
by Baker & Taylor Publisher Services